T0180159

Obesity and Metabolic Surgery

Jürgen Ordemann • Ulf Elbelt

Editors

Obesity and Metabolic Surgery

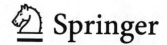

Editors
Jürgen Ordemann
Center for Obesity and
Metabolic Surgery
Vivantes Klinikum Spandau
Berlin, Germany

Ulf Elbelt
Division of Medicine B
University Hospital Ruppin-
Brandenburg
Brandenburg Medical School
Neuruppin, Germany

Endokrinologikum Berlin MVZ
Berlin, Germany

Medical Department
Division of Psychosomatic Medicine
Campus Benjamin Franklin
Charité-Universitätsmedizin Berlin
Corporate Member of Freie
Universität Berlin and Humboldt-
Universität zu Berlin
Berlin, Germany

This book is a translation of the original German edition „Adipositas- und metabolische Chirurgie" by Ordemann, Jürgen, published by Springer-Verlag GmbH, DE in 2017. The translation was done with the help of artificial intelligence (machine translation by the service DeepL.com). A subsequent human revision was done primarily in terms of content, so that the book will read stylistically differently from a conventional translation. Springer Nature works continuously to further the development of tools for the production of books and on the related technologies to support the authors.

ISBN 978-3-662-63229-1   ISBN 978-3-662-63227-7   (eBook)
https://doi.org/10.1007/978-3-662-63227-7

This Springer imprint is published by the registered company Springer-Verlag GmbH, DE, part of Springer Nature.
The registered company address is: Heidelberger Platz 3, 14197 Berlin, Germany

Preface

Isolated cases of pronounced obesity have been found since the early stages of human history. However, obesity has emerged to be a significant health problem over the last 100 years—with unforeseeable consequences for the development of mankind. Obesity is a chronic disease that can shorten life span and lead to various complications such as metabolic syndrome, sleep-related breathing disorders, neoplasm and reduced fertility.

The effect of conservative treatment is usually low and of limited duration. Conservative therapies such as nutritional therapy, physical exercise therapy and behavioural therapy are associated with major challenges for the person concerned. In the case of drug therapy, undesirable effects can also occur. To date, the underlying pathophysiology and genetic predisposition of the affected persons cannot be adequately addressed by conservative therapies and the dramatic environmental changes leading to obesity are also difficult to influence at an individual level.

In contrast, surgical measures can significantly improve the course of obesity. Mortality and morbidity are significantly reduced compared to conservative therapy. In the meantime, obesity surgery and metabolic surgery have become established forms of therapy for obesity and its complications. Due to insufficient information, however, patients who are affected and their therapists still have considerable concern. In addition, health insurance companies also have strong reservations. In comparison to other countries, obesity surgery is still very rarely performed in Germany.

Our practice-oriented textbook is mainly for surgeons who would like to familiarize themselves with the indications, surgical procedures, metabolic interventions, risks and aftercare of obesity surgery. An interdisciplinary approach in the treatment of people with obesity and associated secondary diseases is of particular importance. For this reason, nutritional medicine, internal medicine and psychosomatic issues are featured in this textbook in detail. Our textbook is also intended to help guide nutritional physicians, internists, general practitioners and members of the professional groups involved in the treatment of obesity. We intend to provide practical knowledge for the care of obese patients and to improve the understanding of prevention, complications and aftercare of bariatric surgery for these different professional groups.

Many people contributed their expertise to the development of this textbook. First, our thanks go to the authors of the different chapters. We would also like to thank Dr. Fritz Kraemer and the team at Springer. We would like to particularly thank our editor Heidrun Schoeler for her cooperation and commitment.

We hope that this textbook will be helpful to professionals who are involved in the treatment of obesity and that it will encourage them to provide an interdisciplinary approach to their patients.

Jürgen Ordemann
Berlin, Germany

Ulf Elbelt
Berlin, Germany
January 2021

Contents

Contributors

H. Berger Practice for Nutritional Therapy and Counselling, Lebenswert Essen, Berlin, Germany

J. Birnbaum Department of Anaesthesiology and Intensive Care Medicine, Campus Charité Mitte and Campus Virchow-Klinikum, Charité—Universitätsmedizin Berlin, Berlin, Germany

C. Denecke Department of Surgery, Campus Charité Mitte and Campus Virchow-Klinikum, Charité-Universitätsmedizin Berlin, Berlin, Germany

O. Dietl Dr. Lubos Kliniken, Obesity Center Munich, Klinik Bogenhausen, Munich, Germany

A. Dietrich Clinic and Polyclinic for Visceral, Transplantation, Thoracic and Vascular Surgery, University Hospital Leipzig AöR, Leipzig, Germany

T. Dziodzio Department of Surgery, Campus Charité Mitte and Campus Virchow-Klinikum, Charité—Universitätsmedizin Berlin, Berlin, Germany

U. Elbelt Division of Medicine B, University Hospital Ruppin-Brandenburg, Brandenburg Medical School, Neuruppin, Germany

T. Hofmann Department for Psychosomatic Medicine, Charité-Universitätsmedizin Berlin, Berlin, Germany

T. P. Hüttl Dr. Lubos Kliniken, Obesity Center Munich, Klinik Bogenhausen, Munich, Germany

C. A. Jacobi Adiposity Center Wesseling, Wesseling, Germany

H. Köhler Herzogin Elisabeth Hospital, Obesity Center, Germany

J. Mall Hospital Nordstadt KRH, Clinic for General, Visceral, Vascular and Bariatric Surgery, Hannover, Germany

C. Menenakos Klinikum Barnim GmbH, Eberswalde, Germany

J. Mühlsteiner Clinical Department of General Surgery, University Hospital Graz, Austria

J. Ordemann Center for Obesity and Metabolic Surgery, Vivantes Klinikum Spandau, Berlin, Germany

P. Stauch Dr. Lubos Kliniken, Obesity Center Munich, Klinik Bogenhausen, Munich, Germany

A. Stengel Department of Psychosomatic Medicine and Psychotherapy, University Hospital Tübingen, Tübingen, Germany

Department for Psychosomatic Medicine, Charité—Universitätsmedizin Berlin, Berlin, Germany

R. Weise Adipositas-Zentrum Nord-West, St. Marien-Hospital, Friesoythe, Germany

Obesity

J. Ordemann, U. Elbelt, A. Stengel, and T. Hofmann

Contents

© Springer-Verlag GmbH Germany, part of Springer Nature 2022
J. Ordemann, U. Elbelt (eds.), *Obesity and Metabolic Surgery*,
https://doi.org/10.1007/978-3-662-63227-7_1

1.1 Classification of Obesity

J. Ordemann and U. Elbelt

Obesity is defined as an increase in fat mass beyond the normal level with unfavourable effects on health. Usually, the Body Mass Index (BMI) is used to classify overweight and obesity. It is the quotient of body weight and squared height (unit: kg/m^2). According to the WHO classification, overweight (preadiposity) is defined by a BMI of 25.0–29.9 kg/m^2. A BMI of ≥ 30 kg/m^2 and above is considered as obesity, which is subdivided into different degrees of severity (◻ Table 1.1).

The BMI is easy to determine and is therefore a practical approach for a quick assessment of the nutritional status. However, BMI classification is not sufficient for the assessment of the burden of obesity; in particular, the pattern of fat distribution has to be taken into account. A particular high risk for the development of cardiovascular and metabolic diseases is present when the "visceral" fat mass increases in comparison to the subcutaneous fat mass. Abdominal (visceral or also central) obesity is also known as "apple shaped". In subcutaneous (gluteal-femoral or peripheral) obesity, there is an increase in fat mass mainly in the region of the hips and thighs; this form is also known as "pear type". The fat distribution pattern can be determined by circumfer-

ential measurements. If the waist-to-hip ratio is greater than 0.85 for women and greater than 0.90 for men, abdominal obesity is present; if the ratio is less, peripheral obesity is assumed.

1.2 "Globesity": The Current Pandemic

No other disease is spreading as strongly and as rapidly as obesity. The World Health Organization WHO refers to a worldwide epidemic of obesity. Obesity is no longer just a disease of the individual, but also socioeconomic problem for communities. In some countries, normal weight has now become the exception, and overweight and obesity are the rule. The consequences are catastrophic. Mortality is increasing and life expectancy is falling. As a result of obesity, not only diabetes mellitus type 2, cardiovascular diseases, sleep-related respiratory disorders, tumour diseases and infertility are on the rise, but also epigenetic changes caused by obesity will have an impact on future generations.

National and international health authorities are aware of this challenge and the global threat, but the necessary political consequences are still insufficient. The economic burden of the obesity epidemic on public health services is already considerable. In a study from 2015, the research unit of the management consultancy McKinsey estimates the costs of the obesity epidemic at approximately 1.6 trillion Euros per year—comparable to the costs caused by war and terror.

Epidemiological data on overweight and obesity impressively describe the dramatic increase. In large parts of the world, such as in Asia, the disease is progressing rapidly; as children and adolescents are particularly affected, the dynamics appear particularly threatening.

In a recently published analysis in the Lancet (Ng et al. 2014; ◻ Fig. 1.1) it is stated that currently one third of the world population is overweight or obese. The total number of all overweight or obese people worldwide has risen from 875 million in 1980 to 2.1 bil-

◻ **Table 1.1** Classification of overweight according to body mass index

Classification	BMI (kg/m²)	Risk of secondary disease
Underweight	<18.5	
Normal weight	18.5–24.9	
Overweight/ preadiposity	25.0–29.9	Slightly elevated
Obesity grade I	30.0–34.9	Increased
Obesity grade II	35.0–39.9	Significantly increased
Obesity grade III	≥40	Highly increased

1

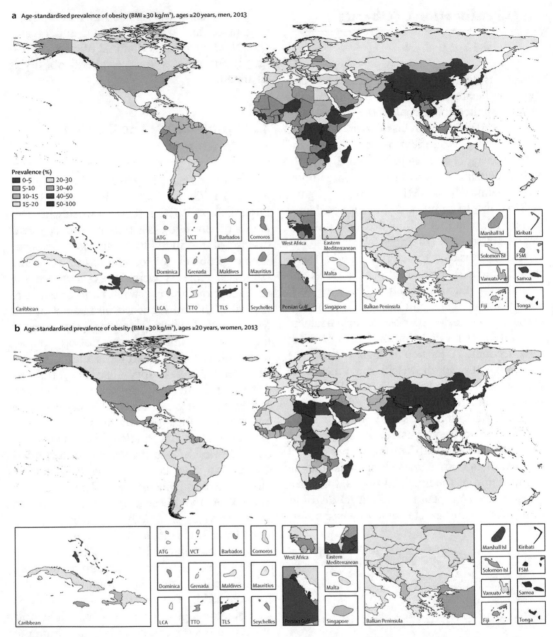

◻ Fig. 1.1 Age-standardised prevalence of obesity (BMI ≥ 30 kg/m², age ≥20 years) in 2013: **a** men, **b** women. (From Ng et al. 2014, with kind permission)

lion. Furthermore, the number of overweight people is growing much faster than the world population as a whole. According to this study from Washington, most obese people live in a total of 10 countries. These include the USA, China, India and Germany.

The incidence of obesity reaches extreme levels in the southern and western Pacific islands. In Micronesia, Tonga or the Cook Islands, about 70% of the population is obese.

According to the Study on Adult Health in Germany (Studie zur Gesundheit

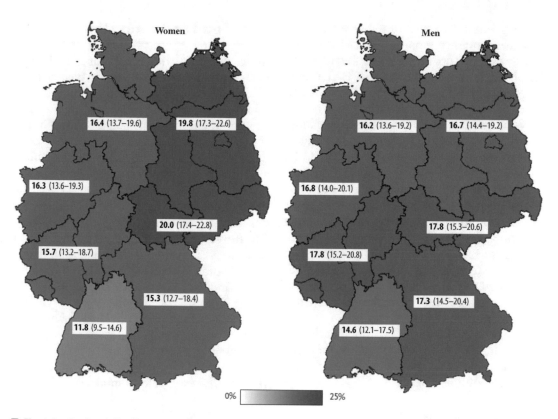

◘ Fig. 1.2 Regional distribution of obesity among women and men. (Robert Koch Institute 2014, with kind permission)

Erwachsener in Deutschland, DEGS) by the Robert Koch Institute (2008–2011), 67% of men and 53% of women in Germany are overweight or obese (◘ Fig. 1.2). 23% of men in Germany have a BMI above 30 kg/m² and are therefore obese. In 1998, the figure was 19%. The prevalence for women in Germany is 24%. Comparable data are found in the Health Survey (Gesundheitsbefragung, GEDA) of the Robert Koch Institute from the year 2012, according to which 17% of men and 16% of women are obese.

In particular, the situation of children and adolescents has worsened considerably in Germany over the recent years. According to the study on the Health of Children and Adolescents in Germany (Studie zur Gesundheit von Kindern und Jugendlichen in Deutschland, KIGGS, 2003–2009)—also by the Robert Koch Institute—15% of children and adolescents are overweight or obese, which corresponds to approximately 800,000 obese children and adolescents.

1.3 Why Are We Getting More and More Obese? Etiology and Pathophysiology

J. Ordemann and U. Elbelt

Obesity is a chronic disease. It is based on a disturbed energy balance with a predominance of energy intake through food with insufficient energy expenditure.

The total energy expenditure consists of resting energy expenditure, the thermic effect of food, cold-induced thermogenesis and activity energy expenditure. The latter can be further divided into exercise-related activity thermogenesis (EAT) and non-exercise activity thermogenesis (NEAT). In obese people, the resting energy expenditure accounts for about 70% of the total energy expenditure; this component cannot be influenced deliberately and is mainly determined by age, sex and body weight. The percentage share of activity energy expenditure decreases with increasing obesity (approx. 26% of the total energy expenditure in obese people with grade III obesity), whereas the share of EAT is only marginal at best. In this respect, everyday and spontaneous physical activity in obese people plays an important role in weight regulation. An additional role in thermogenesis is taken by the so-called brown adipose tissue (BAT). In contrast to white adipose tissue, this leads to energy expenditure in the form of heat. The brown adipose tissue contains a high number of mitochondria whose respiratory chain is "uncoupled". The brown adipose tissue initially described in newborns is also found to a lesser extent in adults. Experimental studies showed that the activity of brown adipose tissue decreases significantly with increasing body weight.

There are numerous factors that favour obesity (■ Fig. 1.3); taken together, they lead to a disturbance of the energy balance. They are briefly outlined below.

1.3.1 Food and Eating Habits

Since the industrial revolution, food composition and eating habits have changed significantly. While a long-lasting reduced food intake leads to a reduction of the resting energy expenditure, an increased food intake ("calorie intoxication") does not lead to an increase of the energy expenditure; this imbalance reflects a bias of the energy balance.

Today, food can be purchased permanently and for a cheap price. In addition, it has also become increasingly energy dense. The increase in calorie intake is exemplified by data from the National Health and Nutrition Examination Survey (NHANES) II (1976–1980) and NHANES III (1988–1991) in the USA. During the period 1976–1991, men increased their energy intake by about 5%, women by an average of 15%. In this respect the energy intake of women has converged to that of men. Other countries showed comparable increases in calorie intake (■ Fig. 1.4).

■ **Fig. 1.3** Compilation of factors favouring obesity

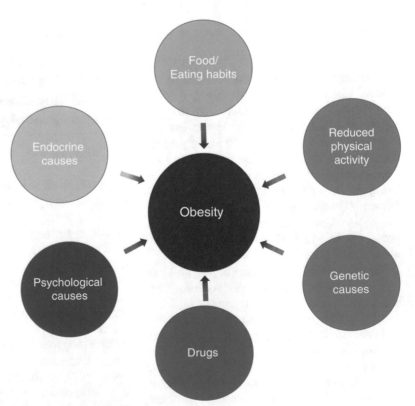

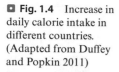 **Fig. 1.4** Increase in daily calorie intake in different countries. (Adapted from Duffey and Popkin 2011)

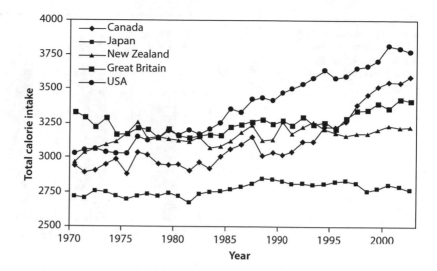

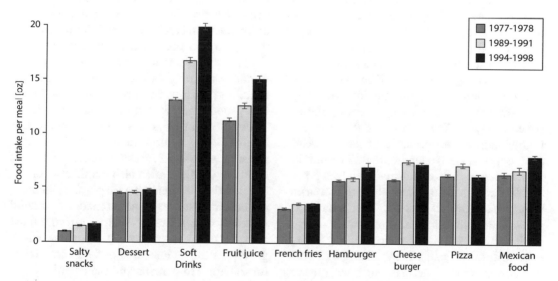

Fig. 1.5 Increase in portion sizes from 1977–1998. (Adapted from Nielsen and Popkin 2003)

An increase in the number of daily meals and portion sizes between the time periods 1977–1978 and 2003–2006 led to an increase in total daily energy intake of 570 kcal. This increase is mainly due to sugar consumption in the form of soft drinks and fruit juices (■ Fig. 1.5). In addition, traditional nutritional patterns are increasingly being abandoned and replaced by more frequent meals outside the home and the increased consumption of convenience foods with high energy density.

1.3.2 Lack of Physical Activity

In addition to the changes in dietary habits described above, the energy expenditure due to physical activity is dramatically declining. As an example of the traditional lifestyle, the exercise behaviour of the Amish religious community in the USA (Amish People) was investigated. There, women had an average daily number of 15,000 steps, men averaged 21,000 steps per day. In a population-based study of

1

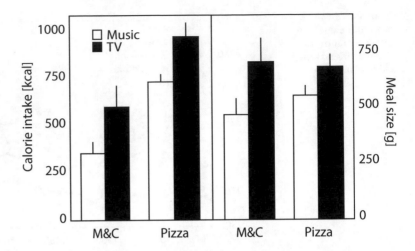

◻ Fig. 1.6 Television consumption is accompanied by an increase in calorie intake. (Adapted from Blass et al. 2006)

physical activity in Colorado—representative of the Western lifestyle—the average number of steps per day was 6600 for women and just over 7000 for men. Thus, the number of steps has fallen to about a third under modern living conditions. This reduction corresponds to a daily deficit of about 500 kcal of energy expenditure. Furthermore, the population-based study by Wyatt et al. (2005) showed a highly significant correlation between weight category and daily step number. The number of steps per day in normal-weight persons (7259) decreased continuously with increasing weight category; it was 6704 for overweight persons and 4866 for obese persons.

Furthermore, the decrease in energy expenditure is caused by changing working conditions—a decrease in hard physical work due to mechanisation and an increase in office work—as well as changes in leisure time behaviour in the form of TV and computer consumption. ◻ Figure 1.6 illustrates that changed media behaviour leads not only to a decrease in physical activity but even to an increase in energy intake.

1.3.3 Genetic Causes

For the genetic predisposition of obesity development, various genetic variants have been identified in genome-wide association studies (e.g. in the FTO gene). However, these individual variants in themselves explain only small increases in weight, so that a polygenic predisposition can be assumed. So far, genetic testing has not been of high clinical relevance.

The monogenetic forms of obesity with mutations mainly in the leptin-melanocortin signalling pathway must be distinguished from the genetic predisposition described above. These forms of obesity are a rarity and occur in childhood. A more detailed description is given in ▶ Sect. 5.2. Furthermore, syndromic forms of obesity which also manifest in childhood and are associated with physical stigmas, endocrine disorders and sometimes mental retardation (e.g. Prader-Willi syndrome) must also be taken into account. In these cases, genetic testing is indicated and can be a relief for the affected persons and their families.

1.3.4 Psychological Causes

Psychosocial factors reinforce the development of obesity favoured by current dietary and exercise habits and should be adequately considered both in diagnosis and therapy.

A change in family structures and occupational demands—work intensification on the one hand and the burden of unemployment on the other—lead to an increased stress perception and social isolation with psychological effects that can further intensify the changes in food intake and eating behaviour described above. Self-stigmatisation of obesity as well as stigmatisation by the social environment represent a further burden. A detailed description of obesity-related mental stressors and mental illness is given in ▶ Sect. 1.5.

1.3.5 Endocrine Causes

The effect of (sub-) clinical hypothyroidism on weight development is usually overestimated. The distinction between hypercortisolism (Cushing's syndrome) and common obesity is often difficult even for an experienced clinician. Although hypercortisolism is also rare in obese people, the individual benefit of early detection is high, so that testing for hypercortisolism should be performed at low-threshold. More on this in ▶ Sect. 5.2.

1.3.6 Drugs Promoting Weight Gain

Numerous drug classes promote weight gain. In particular, tricyclic antidepressants stimulate appetite and hunger and can there-fore lead to considerable weight gain. Other weight gain promoting drugs are neuroleptics, glucocorticoids, insulins, sulfonylureas and thiazolidinediones.

1.4 Regulation of Hunger and Satiety in Obesity

A. Stengel

Contrary to the earlier assumption of a primary regulation of hunger and satiety at a central level in the brain, the current state of knowledge points primarily to a peripheral production of food-regulatory messenger substances. The main sources of these hormones are specialized cells in the gastrointestinal tract. The hormones act via the so-called gut-brain axis (◘ Fig. 1.7) to signal hunger or satiety in the brain and to keep body weight constant in a physiological way. In the following, these regulatory mechanisms, the pathophysiological changes of these systems in obesity as well as psychological factors are described in more detail.

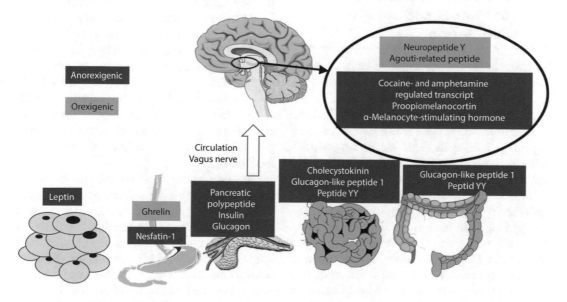

◘ **Fig. 1.7** Hormones, which are involved in the regulation of food intake via the gut-brain axis

1.4.1 Definition of Hunger and Satiety

The German language primarily distinguishes hunger (a sensation localised in the stomach area which causes the need for food intake; this can be further distinguished from appetite, which causes the same desire but can arise in the absence of hunger) from satiety (absence/disappearance of the need for food intake). The English language allows for a more complex understanding of satiety: on the one hand "satiation" (leads to the termination of a meal), on the other hand "satiety" (leads to a subsequent delay between meals). Both together contribute to the termination of the meal and prevent the next meal from being started immediately. In order to make these quantities measurable, the determination of the microstructure of food intake—i.e., meal size, duration, eating speed, interval between meals—is state of the art in animal research as well as in studies on humans.

1.4.2 Peripheral Mediators of Hunger and Satiety Regulation

During the gastrointestinal passage ingested food comes into contact with the gastric mucosa for a longer period of time. Specialised endocrine cells are located in the gastric mucosa, which secrete food-regulating peptides. Such cells (here called enteroendocrine cells) are also found further distal in the intestinal tract. Their hormonal release is induced by nervous stimuli, which in turn are triggered by stretch receptors that react to changes of volume and pressure in the stomach and intestine. Gut chemosensors also play a role: they detect food components and also cause neuronal activation. Recently, bile acids have also been attributed a function in the regulation of food intake; corresponding receptors have recently been identified in the enteric nervous system. In the following, the enteroendocrine cells and their peptide products will be described.

Ghrelin

Ghrelin was discovered in the stomach in 1999 and is the only known peripherally produced and centrally acting hormone that stimulates food intake. Ghrelin is produced in the X/A-like cell (called P/D1 cell in humans). The main source of production seems to be the stomach, as circulating ghrelin levels in patients after gastrectomy fall by 65%. The hormone carries a unique modification in the form of a fatty acid (acyl group) at the third amino acid. This modification is essential for binding to the ghrelin receptor. Recently, the enzyme that catalyses this acylation was identified and named ghrelin-O-acyltransferase (GOAT). Since GOAT is the only enzyme that controls this change, it could be a target molecule for the drug treatment of obesity.

Ghrelin was recognized early on as a food-regulating peptide that has a food-stimulating (orexigenic) function. The meal-dependent regulation supports the assumption that ghrelin is a physiological regulator of food intake. Circulating ghrelin levels rise before food intake and fall again after food intake. Interestingly, the presentation of images with food (during the cephalic phase) also leads to a change in ghrelin levels. Besides these directly food-associated changes, fasting leads to an increase in both the production and release of ghrelin. The ghrelin-activating enzyme GOAT also increases under fasting conditions both in the stomach and in the blood. This could contribute to an increased acylation/activation of ghrelin with the aim of stimulating food intake.

In addition to these short- and medium-term influences on ghrelin, long-term changes in body weight also lead to adaptive changes in ghrelin levels. While ghrelin circulates in higher levels under conditions of cachexia/anorexia, obese people show low ghrelin concentrations in the blood. This could be an attempt by the body to adapt in order to counteract further weight loss in the case of underweight or a further increase in body weight in the case of obesity. However, it should be noted that the postprandial decline of ghrelin in obesity is also attenuated. This could contribute to a reduced feeling of satiety after food intake and thus play a pathophysiological role in the maintenance of obesity.

Nesfatin-1

Interestingly, another hormone has recently been described in the ghrelin-producing cells of the stomach. Nesfatin-1 was initially identified in the rat brain as an inhibitor of food intake (anorexigenic), but was detected shortly thereafter in significantly higher concentrations in the stomach. Here the peptide was localized in the same endocrine X/A-like cells as ghrelin, but in different vesicle populations. This co-localisation led to the concept of a differential regulation of food intake by this specific endocrine cell in the stomach: While food intake is stimulated by the release of ghrelin, it can be inhibited by the release of nesfatin-1. Like ghrelin, nesfatin-1 is also regulated by food intake. A fasting period of 24 h led to a decrease in circulating levels of nucleobindin-2 (NUCB2, the precursor protein of nesfatin-1) and nesfatin-1 in rats—an effect that could be reversed by feeding the animals. A change in nesfatin-1 levels was also observed under long-term changes in body weight: While anorexic patients showed lower levels, obese patients showed higher circulating NUCB2/nesfatin-1 concentrations. This change is opposite to that of ghrelin, which further supports the hypothesis that these two peptides differentially influence food intake. However, it has to be clarified to what extent nesfatin-1, as described in the animal model, also inhibits food intake in humans and thus represents a potential target molecule in pharmacological obesity therapy.

Cholecystokinin

Cholecystokinin (CCK) is produced in the enteroendocrine I-cells of the duodenum and jejunum and is released postprandially. CCK mediates a variety of digestive functions: the contraction of the gallbladder (which gave the hormone its name), the stimulation of exocrine pancreatic secretion, the increase in gastric accommodation and the reduction of food intake. These effects are mediated by two receptors—CCK1 and CCK2—with the peripheral reduction of food intake apparently being primarily induced by CCK1. CCK2 is primarily expressed in the brain, where it is involved in mediating the anorexigenic effect of CCK. The release of CCK is attenuated in obese people, which could lead to a reduced reduction in food intake. In addition to these short-term changes in food intake, CCK also appears to be involved in the regulation of body weight. For example, CCK knockout animals show a reduced body weight (despite unchanged food intake) due to impaired fat absorption in the intestine and increased energy expenditure. These changes led to a resistance to the development of diet-induced obesity and make CCK an interesting substance for pharmacologically influencing/treating obesity.

Pancreatic Polypeptide

Pancreatic polypeptide is released from pancreatic PP cells located within the endocrine islets of Langerhans. This hormone is released after meals, with an increase in circulating levels lasting several hours. In addition to this short-term regulation by food intake, the circulating levels of pancreatic polypeptide are also determined by body weight: While anorexic patients showed significantly increased levels, these were reduced in obese patients. Since pancreatic polypeptide reduces food intake, the changes described above could cause the pathologically altered body weight to be maintained or increased.

Peptide YY

Peptide YY (PYY) is produced by the endocrine L-cells of the distal intestinal tract (decrease from the rectum to the jejunum) and is secreted after a meal. PYY_{1-36} represents the biologically active form, which is activated by dipeptidyl peptidase 4 by cleavage and binds to Y_1 and Y_2 receptors. An anorexigenic role of PYY in the regulation of food intake was postulated—an effect that was also observed in obese patients. However, it should be noted that several follow-up studies could not confirm this effect, so that the role of PYY in the regulation of food intake is considered uncertain or should at least be viewed critically. The body weight-dependent regulation of PYY has also not yet been clarified conclusively.

1

Glucagon-Like Peptide 1

Glucagon-like peptide 1 (GLP-1) is also produced in the enteroendocrine L-cells of the small intestine and is released postprandially. Interestingly, the expectation of a meal also leads to an increase in circulating GLP-1 levels, so that stimulation of the release already in the cephalic phase is obvious. GLP-1 also led to a reduction in food intake, an effect that was also observed in obese patients. In addition, repetitive subcutaneous injections of GLP-1 resulted in a decrease in body weight in obese patients. In addition to its anorexigenic property, GLP-1 leads to an inhibition of glucagon secretion and stimulates insulin secretion (so-called incretin effect). Incretin-based therapies already play a major role in diabetes therapy and are now also approved for the medical therapy (see also ▶ Sect. 2.3).

Leptin

For a long time, adipose tissue was considered to be solely a storage place for energy. According to current knowledge, this tissue is also endocrine active and produces adipokines. The most prominent representative of this group is leptin, which is produced in adipose tissue in dependence of fat mass. Circulating leptin levels also increase with increasing body weight. Leptin leads mainly to a negative energy balance by reducing food intake and by increasing energy expenditure. In addition, leptin is involved in the long-term regulation of body weight. Despite the pronounced effects of leptin administration on body weight regulation in children with congenital leptin deficiency, the effects of such leptin administration in common obesity are small due to the already high leptin levels and the resulting reduced leptin sensitivity. Therefore, leptin does not appear to be a suitable target molecule for the drug treatment of common obesity.

Hormones, which are primarily involved in the regulation of glucose metabolism, also influence food intake and are described below.

Insulin

In addition to the well-described effect on glucose metabolism (leading to a reduction in blood glucose levels via various mechanisms), insulin produced in the beta cells of the endocrine pancreas is also involved in the regulation of food intake and energy balance. The circulating insulin levels correlate—similar to leptin—with the body mass index. In the animal model, the central application of insulin acutely led to a reduction in food intake and, with repetitive administration, also to a reduced increase in body weight. Since insulin can cross the blood-brain barrier, such a regulation is also conceivable under physiological conditions. Whether insulin also plays a significant role in the regulation of hunger and satiety as well as in the regulation of body weight in humans needs further investigation.

Glucagon

Glucagon is produced in the alpha cells of the islets of Langerhans of the endocrine pancreas and, like GLP-1 described above, is a member of the glucagon family. In addition to its well characterized effect on glucose homeostasis (elevation of blood glucose levels in hypoglycemia), glucagon also plays a role in the regulation of food intake. A reduction of food intake by peripheral administration of glucagon has been reported early on, an effect that is likely to be transmitted via the vagus nerve and may be associated with a reduction in gastric emptying. Inhibition of the orexigenic hormone ghrelin may also play a role in mediating the inhibition of food intake by glucagon. In addition, glucagon stimulates thermogenesis and thus leads to an increase in energy expenditure, which could contribute to the observed reduction in body weight in humans after repeated administration of glucagon. Interestingly, glucagon also stimulates the activity of brown adipose tissue in animal models. It has to be clarified whether this signalling pathway is also relevant for the glucagon-induced increase in energy expenditure in humans. In the context of these effects a therapeutic impact of glucagon is discussed, especially in combination with GLP-1 as a dual or co-agonist.

1.4.3 Signalling from the Periphery to the Brain

Various peptide hormones act directly on the brain, in particular on hypothalamic structures. They are often transported across the blood-brain barrier or in the area of the circumventricular organs which is characterized by a lack of the blood-brain barrier. Furthermore, signals are transmitted via the vagus nerve. The vagus nerve has numerous receptors for peptide hormones and transmits the neuronal signal to higher regulatory centres, particularly in the hypothalamus, via the brain stem.

1.4.4 Central Nervous Signal Integration

Specific regions in the brain integrate the signals coming from the periphery and mediate weight-increasing (orexigenic) or weight-reducing (anorexigenic) effects. The most important of these are the nucleus tractus solitarius in the brain stem and various nuclei in the hypothalamus, especially the nucleus arcuatus (in humans called nucleus infundibularis, but in literature often referred to as nucleus arcuatus) and the nucleus paraventricularis. In the nucleus arcuatus two populations of neurons can be distinguished: One contains neuropeptide Y and agouti-related peptide, two strongly orexigenic signals, and the other co-expresses cocaine and amphetamine regulated transcript (CART) and proopiomelanocortin, both of which have anorexic effects. Proopiomelanocortin is also a precursor protein for other biologically active peptides, including α melanocyte-stimulating hormone, which itself also has anorexic effects. These signals are transferred via projections from the nucleus arcuatus to other nuclei, in particular the nucleus paraventricularis. Next to pharmacological interventions on these central signalling pathways other interventions such as deep brain stimulation represent promising strategies for obesity therapy.

1.4.5 Psychological Constructs

The regulatory mechanisms mentioned above are classically attributed to the homeostatic control of hunger and satiety. This has long been contrasted with the so-called hedonic control of hunger and satiety, which is influenced by reward system, desire and palatability of food. Today, these different systems are perceived less isolated and there is increasing evidence for the involvement of the peptide outlined above in both systems. Various psychological constructs of eating behaviour have been developed considering these influencing factors. These include:
- the food responsiveness (interest in food),
- the liking of food (enjoyment),
- the satiation response (e.g. leaving food on the plate),
- eating in the absence of hunger,
- the relative reinforcing value of food (this describes the effort to gain access to food opposed to the effort to achieve other rewards, such as reading a book)
- the disinhibition of eating (e.g. increased eating in social situations) and
- impulsiveness and self-control.

It is important to note that these constructs overlap and cannot be viewed independently of each other. They can be studied under specialised study conditions and with the help of questionnaires and allow a better characterisation of eating behaviour under various metabolic conditions.

1

> **Conclusion**
> A large number of hormones is involved in the regulation of hunger and satiety. Most of them come from the gastrointestinal tract and act via the gut-brain axis on the brain stem and hypothalamus to signal hunger or satiety. Interestingly, so far only one peripherally produced and centrally acting hormone is known to stimulate food intake: ghrelin. In contrast, there are several anorexigenic hormones (■ Fig. 1.7). Despite increasing knowledge of the regulatory mechanisms of food intake, pharmacological modulation of high-grade obesity has so far been insufficient.

1.5 Secondary Diseases of Obesity

U. Elbelt

The health-related consequences of obesity are numerous. In addition to joint and pulmonary diseases, the unfavourable influence of cardiovascular risk factors such as diabetes mellitus type 2, arterial hypertension and dyslipidaemia are of decisive importance. Furthermore, the risk of developing carcinomas is also increased in the presence of obesity. The life expectancy of obese people is shortened. In 40-year-old obese people, for example, it is reduced by about 7 years. The increased mortality is mostly due to cardiovascular diseases and a higher prevalence of malignancies.

1.5.1 Metabolic Syndrome

For the extent of secondary diseases of obesity, not only the fat mass, but above all the distribution of fat tissue plays a decisive role. In comparison to subcutaneous fat deposits, for example in the buttock and thigh area, the abdominal (or visceral) fat distribution is an essential factor in the development of insulin resistance. Insulin resistance is defined as an impaired response of the body to insulin that leads to reduced glucose uptake in the muscles and reduced hepatic glycogen synthesis. The resulting increased glucose supply to the liver maintains these pathophysiological changes

by increasing hepatic de novo lipogenesis. The joint occurrence of cardiovascular risk factors such as impaired glucose tolerance or diabetes mellitus type 2, dyslipidemia (with reduced HDL cholesterol and increased triglycerides) and arterial hypertension with abdominal obesity as a result of insulin resistance is called metabolic syndrome.

However, the metabolic syndrome has not yet been uniformly defined. At a consensus conference of the International Diabetes Federation (IDF), a standardization of these definitions was carried out (■ Table 1.2). In

■ **Table 1.2** Diagnostic criteria of the metabolic syndrome according to the consensus conference of the International Diabetes Federation (IDF)

Criteria	Values
Presence of central (abdominal or visceral) **obesity** and at least two more of the following criteria	Abdominal girth[a] of European men ≥94 cm, of European women ≥80 cm
Triglycerides	>150 mg/dl (1.7 mmol/L) or specific trigylceride-lowering medication
HDL cholesterol	<40 mg/dl (1.03 mmol/L) for men, <50 mg/dl (1.29 mmol/L) for women or specific HDL-raising medication
High blood pressure	Systolic ≥130 mmHg and/or diastolic ≥85 mmHg or specific antihypertensive medication
Fasting plasma glucose	≥100 mg/dl (5.6 mmol/L) or diagnosed diabetes mellitus type 2

[a]With specific reference values of abdominal girth according to ethnicity, whereby from a BMI > 30 kg/m^2 onwards, the presence of abdominal obesity is to be assumed:
– for Arab and African men/women: ≥94 cm/80 cm
– for Asian and Chinese men/women: ≥90 cm/80 cm
– for South and Central American men/women: ≥90 cm/80 cm
– for Japanese men/women: ≥85 cm/90 cm

doing so, different risks for the development of cardiovascular secondary diseases, which are largely determined by ethnic origin, were taken into account.

Other components of the metabolic syndrome are hyperuricemia, impaired fibrinolysis and in women hyperandrogenemia. Patients with a metabolic syndrome must be considered as high-risk cardiovascular patients. Medical treatment of patients with a metabolic syndrome should particularly address dyslipidemia, arterial hypertension and diabetes mellitus type 2.

Practical Tip

The presence of a metabolic syndrome should be documented in order to classify the patient as a cardiovascular high-risk patient.

1.5.2 Diabetes Mellitus Type 2

Numerous epidemiological studies describe abdominal obesity as an important risk factor for the manifestation of type 2 diabetes mellitus. An example is the Nurses' Health Study: This study showed a 6.2-fold increase in the relative risk for the manifestation of diabetes mellitus type 2 with an abdominal girth of >96.4 cm compared to an abdominal girth of <71 cm within 8 years (Carey et al. 1997). Conversely, a moderate weight reduction—in the case of proven insulin resistance, possibly in combination with the intake of metformin in off-label use—can reduce the risk of diabetes manifestation (Knowler et al. 2002; Tuomilehto et al. 2001). Of importance for this interrelation is the secretion of proinflammatory adipokines by the visceral fatty tissue, which leads to an increase in insulin resistance as a major pathogenetic factor of diabetes mellitus type 2.

Table 1.3 shows the diagnostic criteria for diabetes mellitus type 2.

This interrelation does not apply to autoimmune diabetes mellitus type 1 and pancreoprive diabetes mellitus type 3.

Table 1.3 Diagnostic criteria for diabetes mellitus type 2

HbA_{1c} [a]	≥6.5% or ≥48 mmol/L
Random plasma glucose value	≥200 mg/dl (≥11.1 mmol/L)
Fasting plasma glucose value	≥126 mg/dl (≥7.0 mmol/L)
2-h plasma glucose value in an oral glucose tolerance test with 75 g	≥200 mg/dl (≥11.1 mmol/L)

[a]Diseases that lead to a falsification of the HbA_{1c} value have to be taken into account, in particular those with an altered red blood cell lifespan (anaemia, liver and kidney diseases)

1.5.3 Arterial Hypertension

Arterial hypertension is the most common concomitant disease of obesity (Table 1.4). Its prevalence increases up to five times in obese people. Key factors are the increased secretion of angiotensinogen from adipocytes, which is accompanied by activation of the renin-angiotensin-aldosterone system, and an increased tone of the sympathetic nervous system. Again, weight loss leads to a reduction of systolic and diastolic blood pressure.

Practical Tip

Attention has to be paid to the use of sufficiently large cuffs for blood pressure measurement in obese patients, as otherwise incorrectly high blood pressure values will be measured.

1.5.4 Dyslipidemia

There is a well-documented correlation between obesity and altered lipid patterns. The increase in triglycerides with simultaneously decreased HDL-cholesterol is called dyslipidemia. The level of LDL cholesterol is less affected by the extent of obesity, but the composition of LDL cholesterol is altered in

1

◻ Table 1.4 Graduation of arterial hypertension

Blood pressure (mmHg)	High normal	Hypertension grade 1	Hypertension grade 2	hypertension grade 3
Systolic blood pressure	130–139	140–159	160–179	≥180
or				
Diastolic blood pressure	85–89	90–99	100–109	≥110

obesity. This leads to an increase in the highly artherogenic small-dense LDL particles.

1.5.5 Cardiovascular Complications

Obesity is now considered an independent risk factor for heart attack, (diastolic) heart failure (also known as obesity cardiomyopathy) and sudden cardiac death. The risk of cerebrovascular events also increases (probably mainly mediated by concomitant arterial hypertension).

Obesity also leads to disorders of clotting and fibrinolysis. The release of fibrinogen and plasminogen activator-inhibitor-1 (PAI-1) is increased in obesity, resulting in hypercoagulability with increased risk of thrombosis.

1.5.6 Liver Disease

Visceral obesity is considered to be a significant factor for the development of non-alcoholic fatty liver disease. The fatty degeneration of the liver (steatosis hepatis) can progress via inflammatory non-alcoholic steatohepatitis ("non-alcoholic steatohepatits", NASH) to liver cirrhosis and promote the development of hepatocellular carcinoma. Here, too, insulin resistance is regarded as a central pathogenetic factor, so that the liver changes must be regarded as a hepatic manifestation of the metabolic syndrome. The increase of γ-glutamyl-transferase (γ-GT) and alanine-aminotransferase (ALT) as well as—less pronounced—of aspartate-aminotransferase (AST) and alkaline phosphatase (AP) may indicate NASH at an early stage.

1.5.7 Obesity and Sleep-Related Breathing Disorders

Obesity increases the risk of developing a mostly obstructive (but also central or mixed) sleep apnea syndrome (OSA). A neck circumference of more than 43 cm in men or 40.5 cm in women is associated with a significantly increased frequency of nocturnal apneas. Men are four times more frequently affected than women. The leading clinical sign is increased daytime fatigue. Another manifestation is obesity hypoventilation syndrome (OHS), formerly known as "Pickwick's syndrome". It is defined as alveolar hypoventilation with hypercapnia (arterial $pCO_2 \geq 45$ mmHg), mainly during sleep but also in the waking state, with a BMI ≥ 30 kg/m^2, excluding other causes leading to hypoventilation. It often occurs together with obstructive sleep apnea syndrome. The prevalence correlates with the degree of obesity and is given as 3.7/1000 persons for the USA. OHS is considered underdiagnosed, the diagnosis is often made late in the course of acute respiratory insufficiency. Patients predominantly require night-time CPAP ("continuous positive airway pressure") ventilation.

> **Practical Tip**
>
> Obesity and sleep-related breathing disorders are often insufficiently diagnosed. Symptoms should be explicitly asked for in the anamnesis interview. The use of questionnaires can be helpful. Attentive preoperative diagnostics should be carried out to improve the patient's operability by initiating ventilation therapy.

1.5.8 Diseases of the Musculoskeletal System

A common problem is degenerative joint disease, which occurs more frequently and also earlier in obesity. In particular, gonarthrosis and coxarthrosis form an obstacle to the desired increase of physical activity for the treatment of obesity. Furthermore, dorsopathies occur also more frequently. The activation of inflammatory signalling pathways may promote synovial damage.

1.5.9 Malignant Diseases

The carcinoma risk of obese people is increased. For every 5 kg/m^2 increase in BMI, the risk of developing a malignant disease increases by 12–51%, depending on the tumour entity. There is convincing evidence for the more frequent occurrence of colorectal carcinomas, renal cell carcinomas, adenocarcinomas of the esophagus and cardia, and pancreatic carcinomas. The increase in relative risk per 5 kg/m^2 higher BMI is stated to be 18% for colorectal carcinomas; mainly due to the increased risk in men. The extent of insulin resistance also seems to play an additional role. Hyperinsulinemia enhances mitogenic processes by influencing natural cell death (apoptosis) and cell proliferation, probably by binding to the receptor for "insulin-like growth factor 1" (IGF-1R). However, an increase of unbound IGF-1 in serum and tissue as well as effects mediated by elevated leptin levels and inflammation are also described. The reduced secretion of adiponectin with antiproliferative and anti-angiogenic effects in obese patients seems to be of additional importance for the development of malignancies. The increased rate of adenocarcinoma of the oesophagus is thought to be caused by the increased incidence of gastroesophageal reflux in obese patients. An increased incidence of hepatocellular carcinomas due to NASH and of prostate carcinomas is also reported. Women have a higher risk of developing carcinomas of the gallbladder and bile ducts as well as oestrogen-dependent tumours such as breast, endometrial, cervical and ovarian carcinomas. For postmenopausal breast carcinoma, an increase of 12% in the relative risk per 5 kg/m^2 higher BMI is stated. The cause seems to be the increased conversion of androgens to oestrogen through increased aromatase activity in visceral fatty tissue. A reduced risk of breast cancer is reported for obese women before menopause. The association of obesity and endometrial carcinoma is more pronounced. Here, a relative risk increase of 50% per 5 kg/m^2 higher BMI is stated. The relative risk of renal cell carcinoma is reported to increase by 24% for men and 34% for women per 5 kg/m^2. So far, there are hardly any reliable findings on the underlying mechanisms for the development of renal cell carcinomas.

1.5.10 Other Obesity-Related Diseases

The occurrence of gastroesophageal reflux disease is also associated with obesity. The increased intra-abdominal pressure in obesity is discussed as causative. Obese people show an increased biliary cholesterol secretion, which significantly promotes the development of chole(cysto)lithiasis—depending on the extent of obesity (for obesity grade I approx. threefold risk, for obesity grade III approx. sevenfold risk)—and increases the incidence of cholesterol stones. Pronounced conservative weight loss or weight reduction achieved by bariatric surgery further increases the risk of gallstone formation. In addition, obese people have an increased risk of developing diverticulitis.

Polycystic ovary syndrome (PCOS) is a common endocrinological disease of premenopausal women and a cause of unfulfilled wish to have a child. It is defined by the occurrence of at least two of the following criteria:

- hyperandrogenism (clinical and/or biochemical),
- menstrual disorder (oligo- or anovulation) and
- polycystic ovaries (ultrasonography).

1

Other causes have to be excluded before the diagnosis is made. Insulin resistance is also a decisive pathogenetic factor for PCOS. The diagnosis of PCOS enables the early identification of patients at high risk of developing a metabolic syndrome. Therapy with metformin in off-label use—combined with a change in diet and increased physical activity—can lead to an attenuation of the clinical manifestations.

In obese women, the risk of gestational diabetes is increased during pregnancy, and there is also a higher rate of complications during childbirth, making caesarean section more often necessary. The newborns of obese mothers have an increased risk of neural tube defects and macrosomia.

In case of pronounced cephalgia, the presence of a pseudotumour cerebri (idiopathic intracranial hypertension) should also be considered and appropriate diagnostic procedures should be initiated. In particular, obese women are affected, and a dreaded complication is the loss of vision caused by papilledema.

1.6 Psychosocial Aspects of Obesity

T. Hofmann

Obesity is higher-than-average associated with mental disorders. In this context, it was often assumed in the past that obesity was caused by mental disorders. Currently, however, the prevailing view is that massive overweight on the one hand and psychological problems on the other hand are interrelated both bi-directionally and multi-causally.

However, the prevalence rates of mental disorders in obese populations with no desire for treatment are not, or only slightly, higher than those of the general population. This changes in populations with a desire for treatment. Here, the more invasive the intended intervention is (nutrition/exercise, medication, surgery), the more pronounced the psychopathology appears to be. In preoperative cohorts the prevalence is higher than in obese patients with a wish of conservative treatment, which illustrates both the considerable psychological comorbidity and the increased suffering of patients seeking bariatric surgery. In up to 73% of all preoperative obesity patients at least one mental illness can be identified in their preoperative life span, and up to 56% of all obesity patients suffer from at least one mental illness at the time of preoperative evaluation. More pronounced psychopathology is often associated with female gender, higher BMI and especially lower socioeconomic status.

In comparison to the data given above, 38% of the German general population reported having suffered from a mental disorder in their lifetime; among obese people who had no intention of undergoing weight loss treatment, the figure was 48%.

Reasons for the higher prevalence of mental disorders in cohorts with a desire for surgical treatment are therefore probably primarily due to patient selection. Due to the indication criteria for surgical intervention, these patients have a higher BMI and—as a result—a higher risk of somatic comorbidities and a higher rate of mental disorders. Furthermore, the proportion of patients who hope that a surgical procedure will provide them with a kind of "quick fix", a quick solution to their entire life situation and thus also to their psychological burden, should not be underestimated.

1.6.1 Stigmatisation of Obese People

Stigma refers to characteristics or attributes of persons that are associated with negative evaluations and discredit the person concerned. Stigmatising attitudes towards obese people due to their body weight are widespread in our society. By attributing them as voracious, lazy, weak-willed or undisciplined, obese people are held individually responsible for their weight. Moreover, overweight is devalued in the context of the culturally hegemonic ideal of slimness. Obese people are therefore often affected by disparaging to aggressive statements in everyday life, in the media, and also in their personal relationships. In addition, they often face disadvantages in educational institutions, in professional life and last but not least in the health care system. The stigmatisation seems to increase to the extent that it is assumed that the overweight is due to individual misconduct.

The effects of everyday stigmatisation are manifested for those affected in the psychological sphere by a negative body image, a lower self-esteem, and increasing social isolation. The latter being associated with an increased risk of depression, anxiety disorders and even suicidal thoughts. In addition, stigmatisation favours hunger pangs and even the occurrence of binge-eating disorders. All these interrelations seem to be even more pronounced for children, especially for girls. Furthermore, there are first indications that stigmatisation due to body weight could also be associated with physiological parameters such as elevated blood pressure and poor blood sugar control.

1.6.2 **Quality of Life**

Health-related quality of life, as part of the overall quality of life, plays a role in assessing the impairment of patients as the immediate life threat of a disease decreases and chronicity increases. Against this background, health-related quality of life is of great importance in assessing the need for treatment and in the choice of treatment methods for obesity. Health-related quality of life is generally worse in obese people than in the general population. Patients who undergo bariatric surgery are reported to have an even worse health-related quality of life than BMI-matched patients who do not wish to undergo surgery. This is probably not insignificant for the desire for surgery, since an operative procedure is often associated with a rapid and marked improvement in general well-being. Obese women seem to be more affected by limited health-related quality of life than obese men.

1.6.3 **Stress**

Stress is generally understood to be the physiological and psychological reactions of an organism to challenging environmental conditions (stressors). While stress can lead to reduced body weight, for example in the context of depression, a connection between chronic stress and obesity has been repeatedly postulated. In this context, psychosocial stress has mostly been understood as a consequence of stigmatisation or disadvantages in everyday life. In fact, especially for higher levels of obesity, there are links between the perception of stress and increased body weight.

The so-called "modern lifestyle" with increasingly less physical activity and better availability of high-calorie and energy-dense food (so-called "comfort food") is primarily blamed for the continued rise in the prevalence of, in particular, high-grade obesity. In this context, the increased stress levels in industrialised countries, for example due to higher work density or the overall increasing demands on the individual when reliable social structures dissolve, are less frequently taken into account as another aspect of modern lifestyle. However, there are now plausible psychobiological concepts that conceive the development of obesity also as an adaptation of the organism to chronic psychosocial stress. Thus, in addition to the hypothalamus-pituitary-adrenal cortex axis, cerebral glucose and insulin metabolism as well as other endocrine signals such as ghrelin could play a decisive role.

1.6.4 **Depression**

Depression is characterized by depressed mood and a reduction in drive and activity. In addition, the ability to feel enjoyment, interest and concentration are reduced. Depression is an independent risk factor for several somatic diseases, and this relationship is well documented, especially for coronary heart disease and diabetes mellitus.

The link between obesity and depression has been repeatedly confirmed. However, it seems to be minimal or even non-existent in cohorts without a desire for treatment. This changes in patients with a desire for treatment. According to a meta-analysis of longitudinal studies, obese people, for example, have a 55% higher risk of developing depression than healthy people; conversely, the probability of developing obesity is 58% higher in people suffering from depression.

> **Practical Tip**
>
> The preoperative diagnosis of depression seems to be associated with less weight loss after bariatric surgery. On the other hand, the depressive symptoms seem to be significantly reduced in the majority of patients after surgery, although in some cases this success may weaken over the following years.

1.6.5 Anxiety Disorders

Anxiety disorders include
1. the generalised anxiety disorder with persistent, quasi "free-floating" fears that are not limited to certain environmental conditions,
2. panic disorder with recurrent severe anxiety attacks that are not limited to a specific situation or circumstances, and
3. phobias, where the fears are caused by clearly defined, actually harmless situations. A frequent phobic disorder, even in obese patients, is the social phobia with the fear of being judged by other people, which leads to the avoidance of social situations.

Anxiety disorders are the most common mental disorders in developed countries. Up to 25% of the population are affected within their lifetime. In addition, anxiety disorders generally have a negative impact on the course of chronic diseases. However, the connection between anxiety disorders and obesity is less clear than that for depression. In a meta-analysis, obese people were found to be 40% more at risk of having a concurrent anxiety disorder. This interrelation seems to increase with higher BMI and is most pronounced in anxiety in the context of post-traumatic stress disorders and social anxiety. No statement can be made about the direction of a possible causality or bidirectionality on the basis of the studies available to date.

1.6.6 Neglect, Abuse and Post-traumatic Stress Disorder

There is a well-established link between child abuse and the development of chronic physical illness. Accordingly, the connection between physical and sexual abuse in childhood and the development of obesity is well established. A meta-analysis showed a 36% increased risk for the development of obesity.

Post-traumatic stress disorder (PTSD) is characterized by psychological reactions that occur against the background of a stressful event with exceptional threat. Typical characteristics are re-experiencing of the traumatic event through intrusive thoughts, nightmares and flashbacks, vegetative hyperexcitability and often pronounced avoidance behaviour. Fifty percent of all patients with PTSD show abdominal obesity. The probability of obesity is significantly higher in these patients than in healthy people. In a German prospective longitudinal study, the risk of developing obesity in women, but not in men, was associated with the presence of manifest or subsyndromal PTSD.

1.6.7 Eating Disorders

Disturbed eating behaviour has often been associated with the development of overweight and obesity. Relevant eating disorders associated with obesity include binge-eating disorder and bulimia nervosa. Binge-eating disorder is defined by eating large quantities of food much faster than usual without a physiological feeling of hunger, associated with a loss of control. At least one attack per week over a period of 3 months is required for diagnosis. In addition, feelings of shame or guilt usually occur as a consequence. In contrast to bulimia nervosa, whose core criterion is also eating attacks, there is no regular compensatory behaviour such as vomiting, taking laxatives or pronounced food restriction.

Binge-eating disorder is the most common eating disorder with a prevalence of about 1–3%. In obese cohorts with a desire for surgical treatment, however, the prevalence is significantly higher at up to 50%, which in turn points to an increased psychological comorbidity in this patient group. In contrast to anorexia and bulimia nervosa, binge-eating disorder also affects men to a relevant extent, accounting for about one third of cases.

In a population-based study in 14 countries, it was shown that 33% of all patients with bulimia nervosa and 42% of all patients with binge-eating disorder are obese. In addition, the proportion of patients with binge-eating disorder seems to increase in higher BMI ranges.

Other unfavourable eating habits relevant for the care of obese patients are

- Night-eating syndrome, which is characterised by an intake of food in the evening or at night,
- Sweet-eating syndrome, characterized by excessive consumption of sweet foods, and
- the so-called "grazing" with a repeated and unplanned intake of small amounts of food between regular meals.

However, these definitions are inconsistent and their character as independent diseases is currently under discussion.

1.6.8 Personality and Personality Disorders

Personality traits can be both protective and risk factors for the development of obesity. For example, obsessive-compulsive disorders can be associated with restrictive eating habits and reduced body weight. In contrast, personality traits such as neuroticism (emotional vulnerability, often associated with anxiety, depression, hostility and annoyance), increased impulsiveness or dependence on rewards have been shown to increase the likelihood of obesity. Neuroticism also appears to be associated with a more frequent occurrence of eating attacks in the context of emotional eating. Reward dependency appears to be associated with binge-eating disorder. In contrast, protective effects have been found for characteristics such as conscientiousness or self-control with regard to increasing body weight.

Eating disorders can also be associated with disorders of affect regulation and impulse control, as found in emotionally unstable personality disorders (so-called borderline personality disorders). The prevalence in various clinical obesity populations varies widely, averaging about 25%. In addition, up to about 30% of all obese patients with a binge-eating disorder appear to have a borderline personality disorder, again with large fluctuations in frequency

1.6.9 Substance Abuse

Alcohol abuse seems to occur in obese patients with a desire for obesity surgery treatment with a frequency comparable to that of the general population. There is currently no reliable interrelation between postoperative weight loss and the development of alcohol abuse. According to the few studies available to date, patients with an alcohol abuse in their preoperative history are apparently at increased risk of relapse after bariatric surgery (and especially after a gastric bypass). This could apply not only to alcohol abuse and addiction, but also to other substance-bound and behavioural addictions.

1.6.10 Suicidal Tendencies

While an increased BMI is associated with the increased incidence of mental disorders, various studies suggest that there is an inverse relationship between increased BMI and the risk of a completed suicide. However, the findings are very inconsistent with regard to the risk of suicide attempts and suicidal thoughts or tendencies, and may depend on subgroup characteristics such as psychological comorbidity, age, gender, and country of origin.

Even if the frequency and severity of psychological problems and illnesses initially decrease significantly after bariatric surgical procedures, the suicide risk after bariatric surgery seems to increase slightly overall. In a review, possible factors that could mediate an increased suicide risk after surgery were discussed. Reasons could be the persistence of somatic comorbidities, insufficient weight loss or the (re)appearance of psychological symptoms. Biological aspects of altered gastrointestinal anatomy, such as increased alcohol sensitivity or postprandial hyperinsulinemic hypoglycaemia, and factors that are difficult to modify, such as genetic variations, are also possible.

1.6.11   Social Inequality

Like other chronic diseases and life expectancy in general, obesity is associated with socioeconomic parameters, with a higher social position being associated with a lower BMI. This correlation is more pronounced in women than in men. In addition, it is interesting to note that studies have shown that a higher prevalence of obesity is associated with more pronounced social injustice in the form of income inequality, but not with the average income of an economy. Furthermore, an American prospective social-epidemiological study showed that moving from one neighbourhood with a high poverty index to another with a low poverty index led to reductions in pronounced obesity and diabetes. Psychosocial stress associated with social disadvantage is commonly cited as the mediating variable for this interrelation.

References

1.1 to 1.3

Blass EM, Anderson DR, Kirkorian HL et al (2006) On the road to obesity: television viewing increases intake of high-density foods. Physiol Behav 88: 597–604

Duffey KJ, Popkin BM (2011) Energy density, portion size, and eating occasions: contributions to increased energy intake in the United States, 1977–2006. PLoS Med 8:e1001050

Ng M, Fleming T, Robinson M et al (2014) Global, regional, and national prevalence of overweight and obesity in children and adults during 1980–2013: a systematic analysis for the Global Burden of Disease Study 2013. Lancet 384:766–781

Nielsen SJ, Popkin BM (2003) Patterns and trends in food portion sizes, 1977–1998. JAMA 289:450–453

Robert Koch-Institut (2008) Lebensphasenspezifische Gesundheit von Kindern und Jugendlichen in Deutschland. Ergebnisse des Nationalen Kinder- und Jugendgesundheitssurveys (KiGGS). Gesundheitsberichterstattung des Bundes. http://www.rki.de/DE/Home/hompage_node.html. (19. April 2016)

Robert Koch-Institut (2014) Übergewicht und Adipositas. Faktenblatt zu GEDA 2012: Ergebnisse der Studie "Gesundheit in Deutschland aktuell 2012". http://www.rki.de/DE/Content/Gesundheitsmonitoring/Gesundheitsberichterstattung/GBEDownloadsB/GEDA12.pdf. (19. April 2016)

Wyatt HR, Peters JC, Reed GW et al (2005) A Colorado statewide survey of walking and its relation to excessive weight. Med Sci Sports Exerc 37:724–730

1.5

Carey VJ, Walters EE, Colditz GA et al (1997) Body fat distribution and risk of non-insulin-dependent diabetes mellitus in women. The Nurses' Health Study. Am J Epidemiol 145:614–619

Knowler WC, Barett-Connor E, Fowler SE et al (2002) Reduction in the incidence of type 2 diabetes with lifestyle intervention or metformin. N Engl J Med 346:393–403

Tuomilehto J, Lindström J, Eriksson JG et al (2001) Prevention of type 2 diabetes mellitus by changes in lifestyle among subjects with impaired glucose tolerance. N Engl J Med 344:1343–1350

Further Reading

1.1 to 1.3

Bassett DR, Schneider PL, Huntington GE (2004) Physical activity in an old order Amish community. Med Sci Sports Exerc 36:79–85

Bleich S, Cutler D, Murray C, Adams A (2008) Why is the developed world obese? Ann Rev Public Health 29:273–295

Briefel RR, McDowell MA, Alaimo K et al (1995) Total energy intake of the US population: the third National Health and Nutrition Examination Survey, 1988–1991. Am J Clin Nutr 62(Suppl. 5):1072S–1080S

Elbelt U, Schuetz T, Hoffmann I et al (2010) Differences of energy expenditure and physical activity patterns in subjects with various degrees of obesity. Clin Nutr 29:766–772

Frayling TM, Timpson NJ, Weedon MN et al (2007) A common variant in the FTO gene is associated with body-mass-index and predisposes to childhood and adult obesity. Science 316:889–894

Lean ME, Han TS, Morrison CE (1995) Waist circumference as a measure for indicating need for weight management. BMJ 311:158–161

McKinsey Global Institute (2014) Overcoming obesity: an initial economic analysis. http://www.mckinsey.com/mgi. (19. April 2016)

Mensink GB, Schienkiewitz A, Haftenberger M et al (2013) Übergewicht und Adipositas in Deutschland: Ergebnisse der Studie zur Gesundheit Erwachsener in Deutschland (DEGS1). Bundesgesundheitsblatt Gesundheitsforschung Gesundheitsschutz 56:786–794

Van Marken Lichtenbelt WD, Vanhommerig JW, Smulders NM et al (2009) Cold-activated brown adipose tissue in healthy men. N Engl J Med 360: 1500–1508

WHO Global InfoBase Team (2005) The SuRF Report 2. Surveillance of chronic disease risk factors: country-level data and comparable estimates. World Health Organization. https://apps.who.int/infobase/Publicfiles/SuRF2.pdf. (19. April 2016)

Wiegand S, Krude H (2015) Monogene und syndromale Krankheitsbilder bei morbider Adipositas. Internist 56:111–120

Wirth A, Hauner H (2013) Adipositas Ätiologie, Folgekrankheiten, Diagnostik, Therapie. Springer, Berlin, Heidelberg

1.4

Hussain SS, Bloom SR (2013) The regulation of food intake by the gut-brain axis: implications for obesity. Int J Obes 37:625–633

Konturek SJ, Konturek JW, Pawlik T, Brzozowski T (2004) Brain-gut axis and its role in the control of food intake. J Physiol Pharmacol 55:137–154

Kumar R, Simpson CV, Froelich CA et al (2015) Obesity and deep brain stimulation: an overview. Ann Neurosci 22:181–188

Rindi G, Leiter AB, Kopin AS, Bordi C, Solcia E (2004) The "normal" endocrine cell of the gut: changing concepts and new evidences. Ann NY Acad Sci 1014:1–12

Schwartz MW, Woods SC, Porte D Jr, Seeley RJ, Baskin DG (2000) Central nervous system control of food intake. Nature 404:661–671

Stengel A, Taché Y (2011) The physiological relationships between the brainstem, vagal stimulation, and feeding. In: Preedy VR, Watson RR, Martin CR (Hrsg) Handbook of behavior, diet and nutrition. Springer, New York, Dordrecht, Heidelberg, London, pp. 817–828

1.5

Alberti KG, Zimmet P, Shaw J (2005) The metabolic syndrome—a new worldwide definition. Lancet 366:1059–1062

Borel JC, Borel AL, Monneret D et al (2012) Obesity hypoventilation syndrome: from sleep-disordered breathing to systemic comorbidities and the need to offer combined treatment strategies. Respirology 17:601–610

Deutsche Gesellschaft für Kardiologie, Deutsche Hochdruckliga e.V. DHL (2013) ESH/ESC Pocket Guidelines. Leitlinien für das Management der arteriellen Hypertonie. http://www.hochdruckliga.de/tl_files/content/dhl/downloads/2014_Pocket-Leitlinien_Arterielle_Hypertonie.pdf. (6. Februar 2016)

Flier JS, Maratos-Flier E, Elbelt U, Scholze JE (2012) Adipositas. In: Longo DL, Fauci AS, Kaspar DL, et al. (Hrsg) Harrisons Innere Medizin, 18. Aufl. ABW Wissenschaftsverlag, Berlin, S 665–672

Haslam DW, James WPT (2005) Obesity. Lancet 366:1197–1209

Kerner W, Brückel J (2015) Definition, Klassifikation und Diagnostik des Diabetes mellitus. Diabetol Stoffwechs 10(Suppl. 2):S98–S101

Kushner RF, Elbelt U, Scholze JE (2012) Diagnostik und Management der Adipositas. In: Longo DL, Fauci AS, Kaspar DL, et al. (Hrsg) Harrisons Innere Medizin, 18. Aufl. ABW Wissenschaftsverlag, Berlin, S 673–681

Mallery RN, Friedmann DI, Liu GT (2014) Headache and the pseudotumor cerebri syndrome. Curr Pain Headache Rep 18:446

Nimptsch K, Pischon T (2014) Adipositas und Krebs. Adipositas 8:151–156

Talmor A, Dunphy B (2015) Female obesity and infertility. Best Pract Res Clin Obstet Gynaecol 29:498–506

1.6

Andersen JR, Aasprang A, Karlsen TI et al (2015) Health-related quality of life after bariatric surgery: a systematic review of prospective long-term studies. Surg Obes Relat Dis 11:466–473

Brandheim S, Rantakeisu U, Starrin B (2013) BMI and psychological distress in 68,000 Swedish adults: a weak association when controlling for an age-gender combination. BMC Public Health 13:68

Dallman MF (2010) Stress-induced obesity and the emotional nervous system. Trends Endocrinol Metab 21:159–165

Danese A, Tan M (2014) Childhood maltreatment and obesity: systematic review and meta-analysis. Mol Psychiatry 19:544–554

de Zwaan M, Enderle J, Wagner S et al (2011) Anxiety and depression in bariatric surgery patients: a prospective, follow-up study using structured clinical interviews. J Affect Disord 133:61–68

Gariepy G, Nitka D, Schmitz N (2010) The association between obesity and anxiety disorders in the population: a systematic review and meta-analysis. Int J Obes 34:407–419

Gerlach G, Herpertz S, Loeber S (2015) Personality traits and obesity: a systematic review. Obes Rev 16:32–63

Herpertz S, Burgmer R, Stang A et al (2006) Prevalence of mental disorders in normal-weight and obese individuals with and without weight loss treatment in a German urban population. J Psychosom Res 61:95–103

Kessler RC, Berglund PA, Chiu WT et al (2013) The prevalence and correlates of binge eating disorder in the World Health Organization World Mental Health Surveys. Biol Psychiatry 73:904–914

Ludwig J, Sanbonmatsu L, Gennetian L et al (2011) Neighborhoods, obesity, and diabetes—a randomized social experiment. N Engl J Med 365:1509–1519

Luppino FS, de Wit LM, Bouvy PF et al (2010) Overweight, obesity, and depression: a systematic review and meta-analysis of longitudinal studies. Arch Gen Psychiatry 67:220–229

Malik S, Mitchell JE, Engel S, Crosby R, Wonderlich S (2014) Psychopathology in bariatric surgery candidates: a review of studies using structured diagnostic interviews. Compr Psychiatry 55:248–259

Mitchell JE, Crosby R, de Zwaan M et al (2013) Possible risk factors for increased suicide following bariatric surgery. Obesity 21:665–672

Mitchell JE, Steffen K, Engel S et al (2015) Addictive disorders after Roux-en-Y gastric bypass. Surg Obes Relat Dis 11:897–905

Moore CJ, Cunningham SA (2012) Social position, psychological stress, and obesity: a systematic review. J Acad Nutr Diet 112:518–526

Mühlhans B, Horbach T, de Zwaan M (2009) Psychiatric disorders in bariatric surgery candidates: a review of the literature and results of a German prebariatric surgery sample. Gen Hosp Psychiatry 31:414–421

Pagoto SL, Schneider KL, Bodenlos JS (2012) Association of post-traumatic stress disorder and obesity in a nationally representative sample. Obesity 20:200–205

Peters A, Kubera B, Hubold C, Langemann D (2013) The corpulent phenotype—how the brain maximizes survival in stressful environments. Front Neurosci 7:47

Pickett KE, Kelly S, Brunner E, Lobstein T, Wilkinson RG (2005) Wider income gaps, wider waistbands? An ecological study of obesity and income inequality. J Epidemiol Community Health 59:670–674

Puhl RM, King KM (2013) Weight discrimination and bullying. Best Pract Res Clin Endocrinol Metab 27:117–127

Rosenbaum S, Stubbs B, Ward PB, Steel Z, Lederman O, Vancampfort D (2015) The prevalence and risk of metabolic syndrome and its components among people with posttraumatic stress disorder: a systematic review and meta-analysis. Metabolism 64:926–933

Conservative Treatment of Obesity

U. Elbelt, H. Berger, and T. Hofmann

Contents

© Springer-Verlag GmbH Germany, part of Springer Nature 2022
J. Ordemann, U. Elbelt (eds.), *Obesity and Metabolic Surgery*,
https://doi.org/10.1007/978-3-662-63227-7_2

2.1 Therapeutic Goals

U. Elbelt

The aim of the therapy is sustainable weight reduction and the prevention or improvement of obesity-related comorbidities and secondary diseases. The high prevalence of obesity is mostly explained by over-nutrition and lack of exercise in the context of the prevailing lifestyle. Accordingly, the interdisciplinary S3 Guidelines of the German Obesity Society (DAG), the German Diabetes Society (DDG), the German Nutrition Society (DGE) and the German Society of Nutritional Medicine (DGEM) from 2014 focus on nutrition, physical exercise and behavioural therapy as the basis of obesity treatment. The basic program aims for weight reduction in the first phase and sustained loss of weight in the second phase. The therapeutic goals should be a weight reduction of >5% of the initial weight for persons with a BMI of 25–35 kg/m^2 within 1 year, and a weight reduction of >10% of the initial weight for persons with a BMI > 35 kg/m^2. Furthermore, for persons with a BMI ≥ 28 kg/m^2 with concomitant risk factors and/or comorbidities (or BMI ≥ 30 kg/m^2) additional drug therapy may be initiated following insufficient weight reduction due to lifestyle changes within 6 months or rapid weight regain after a phase of weight reduction.

2.2 Nutrition Therapy

H. Berger and U. Elbelt

Diets aimed at weight reduction are available in numerous variations. The best known are
- calorie-reduced diet according to the Weight-Watchers principle with calculation of the daily energy intake according to a point system (1 point corresponds to approx. 50 kcal, target: 24–32 points/day, corresponding to 1200–1600 kcal/day)
- fat and energy reduced diets (<30% fats),
- Atkins diet with reduced carbohydrate intake of up to 50 g/day,

- drastic reduction of the daily calorie intake (<1000 kcal) by using regulated formulations (protein-rich drinks with added vitamins and minerals).

An effective nutrition therapy must be adapted to the individual needs of the patient. According to the S3 guidelines of the professional societies, a step-by-step scheme should be followed, which takes this into account. The primary focus of the dietary change is on a reduction of the total calorie intake. In the first stage, a reduction in fat and/or carbohydrate intake alone, especially sugar consumption, can lead to a lower energy intake. In the second stage, a calorie deficit of 500–1000 kcal daily compared to the previous calorie intake should be aimed for by an energy-reduced mixed diet (DGE 2009). The calorie restriction should allow a weight loss of 0.5 kg/week. An energy-reduced mixed diet is characterised by a diet rich in fibre and protein as well as fat-moderated food selection and a high proportion of vegetables (and fruit). The nutrient composition should correspond to the reference values with 50–55% carbohydrates, 30% fat and 15–20% protein of the total energy intake (DGE et al. 2008). At the third or fourth stage, individual meals or all meals can be replaced by regulated formulation drinks.

Three ground-breaking randomised studies have compared the success of different dietary regimes. These studies are therefore described in more detail below:
- With regard to weight reduction, an Israeli study found that a calorie-reduced Mediterranean diet and a carbohydrate but not calorie-reduced diet ("low-carbohydrate diet") were significantly superior to a fat and calorie-reduced diet ("low-fat diet") over a period of 2 years (Shai et al. 2008). These two diets were also superior to the low-fat diet with regard to a favourable influence on the lipid pattern. Common to all diets was the significant initial weight loss until the sixth month of the intervention, followed by a renewed weight gain in the following year (exception: Mediterranean diet) and a subsequent phase of

weight stabilisation, so that the weight loss at the end of the second year of the study was 2.9 ± 4.2 kg for the fat-reduced diet, 4.4 ± 6.0 kg for the Mediterranean diet and 4.7 ± 6.5 kg for the carbohydrate-reduced diet. The participants were characterised by a high level of dietary adherence, which at the end of the second year was still at about 85%. This can certainly also be explained by the way the study was conducted, as the participants were recruited via their place of work and the food in the staff canteens was also specifically labelled.

– A study carried out with a higher number of subjects ($N = 811$) on the effect of diets with different proportions of the macronutrients fat, protein and carbohydrates for the total daily energy intake showed no relevant difference after 2 years with regard to the weight loss achieved (Sacks et al. 2009). Depending on the type of diet, the weight loss was between 3.0 kg (for "low fat, high carb") and 4.0 kg (for "low fat"). One explanation for the only slightly different results in weight development is certainly that the desired differences in the composition of the macronutrients could not be achieved as intended. However, in all the dietary forms investigated, a significant increase in the weight loss achieved was found in relation to the intensity of training (measured by participation in nutritional counselling time units).

– The decisive influence of treatment adherence is impressively demonstrated in a study by Dansinger et al.(2005). In this study over 12 months with 160 participants (average age 49 years, average BMI 35 kg/m^2), who had a BMI above 27 kg/m^2 and at least one other cardiovascular risk factor, the participants were randomly assigned to the following diet forms: Diet according to Ornish with a predominantly vegetarian diet and a reduction of the fat content to 10%, calorie-reduced diet according to the Weight-Watchers principle (see above), carbohydrate-reduced diet according to Atkins (see above) and Zone diet with a macronutrient content as constant as possible (40% carbohydrates, 30%

fats and 30% proteins) of the daily energy intake. In the first 2 months of the study, the participants received four nutritional training sessions of 60 min each. At the end of the study, no difference in daily energy intake was observed between the groups. Likewise, no significant difference was observed for weight loss achieved during one year, which was most pronounced in the "Ornish group" with 3.3 ± 7.3 kg and least pronounced in the "Zone group" with 2.1 ± 4.8 kg. At monthly intervals, the dietary adherence of the participants was assessed for all intervention groups using a scale (no dietary adherence corresponds to 1, perfect dietary adherence corresponds to 10). Initially, the average for all groups was between 6 and 7, but then dropped significantly after 1 month and after 1 year the average was only between 2 and 4. The correlation between weight loss and self-estimated dietary adherence was highly significant regardless of the type of diet.

The latter study shows very well that the sustained motivation to change one's diet is crucial for long-term success.

Practical Tip

The possibility to constantly integrate the change in diet into the patient's everyday life is of special importance. Therefore, the individual nutritional preferences and eating habits of the patient have to be taken into account when making dietary recommendations.

Therapists should have a repertoire of nutritional interventions and adapt them specifically to individual needs.

Very low calorie diets using regulated formulation drinks should only be used for targeted short-term weight loss (e.g. before elective joint replacement). The daily calorie intake should not go below 800 kcal and a sufficient fluid intake of approx. 2.5–3 l daily should be ensured. In addition, the regulated formulation products used should comply with the German Dietary Regulations (§7,

§4a, §21a and Appendices 2, 6, 17), which specify the nutrient composition of "dietary foods" (DGE 2009). Low-calorie diets should not be followed for longer than 12 weeks. Renewed weight gain after the end of the high calorie restriction phase is usually rapid and pronounced.

2.3 Physical Exercise

U. Elbelt

In addition to nutrition therapy, physical exercise has so far been attributed a decisive role in weight reduction by increasing energy consumption. Increased physical exercise alone, however, has at best only a small weight-reducing effect; only the combination with a reduction in caloric intake enables weight loss (Franz et al. 2007). In the interdisciplinary S3 guideline, the following recommendations for physical activity are given:
- For effective weight loss, physical exercise for >150 min/week (with the aim of achieving an energy expenditure of 1200–1800 kcal/week) is recommended.
- Strength training alone is not suitable for weight reduction.
- In the case of grade II or III obesity, activities that are stressful for the musculoskeletal system should be avoided.
- An increase in everyday physical activity should be aimed for.
- Independent of weight reduction, physical activity leads to health benefits.

Before starting physical exercise, contraindications for additional physical activity should be excluded.

Increased physical activity is particularly important for maintaining successful weight loss. If weight loss is achieved by reducing calorie intake, the resting energy expenditure is mainly determined by body weight (▶ Sect. 1.2). After termination of the "diets," which are usually carried out only temporarily, this resulting "energy gap" must be permanently bridged. This can only be achieved by continuing strict calories restriction and/or by increasing thermogenesis through increased physical activity. Possible strategies for closing this "energy gap" are described in detail by Wing and Hill (2001). In their observational study, the behaviour of more than 3000 participants in the National Weight Control Registry (NWCR) in the USA was recorded. The participants had lost an average of 30 kg of weight and were able to maintain this weight loss over an average of 5.5 years. The following behavioural patterns characterise these successful participants with sustained weight control:
- 90% of the participants were able to change their diet permanently and increase their physical activity. The necessity of using both strategies (dietary change and increased physical activity) for sustained weight maintenance is also evident from a meta-analysis that takes into account 80 randomised clinical studies with a total of 26,455 participants and an observation period of at least 1 year (Franz et al. 2007). Thus, the combination of dietary change and increased physical activity was superior to dietary change or increased physical activity alone—apart from additional drug interventions.
- The participants behaved very calorie-restrictively, they had an average caloric intake of only 1381 kcal/day; they also adhered a fat-reduced diet (24% fat, 19% protein, 56% carbohydrates).
- The participants carried out regular self-monitoring with nutrition and physical exercise documentation as well as assessment of body weight (44% daily).
- The participants were able to increase their additional physical activity ("regular planned exercise") to about 2800 kcal/week (corresponding to 1 h of brisk walking per day). The most frequent additional physical activity was walking, followed by cycling, weight training and aerobics.

These findings were also confirmed in a 10-year follow-up analysis (Thomas et al. 2014).

It is important to discuss realistic options for increasing physical activity. Physical activity should be integrated into everyday life through increased leisure activities and active commuting (avoiding transportation). Using pedometers and documenting the daily step count is a useful strategy.

2.4 Lifestyle Change: Psychotherapy and Psychoeducation

T. Hofmann

In addition to the already mentioned causes of obesity, increased body weight is often the result of eating habits that are not adapted to biological and psychosocial needs in the long term. However, individual nutritional (and physical activity) behaviour should not be misinterpreted as weakness of will alone (▶ Sect. 1.5.1), with family members in particular, but also doctors seem to be the most frequent sources of such stigmatisation. The individual eating behaviour, as described in ▶ Sect. 1.2, is rather to be seen as the result of complex genetic, biological-physiological, psychological and socio-cultural factors and may be influenced by medical drug therapy. A psychotherapeutic approach should therefore be focused on psychosocial causes or consequences of obesity. This can include the development of tasks for dealing with stigmatisation and self-esteem problems that often result from stigmatisation, but also interventions to improve stress management, to obtain sustainable social support or to deal with external stimuli that initiate unfavourable eating behaviour. In addition, techniques of self-observation (diet and physical exercise diaries, regularly documented weight control) play an important role. It has to be considered whether the initial therapeutic goal should not be achievement of weight reduction, but rather improvement of overall quality of life.

In any case, realistic weight goals should be defined at the beginning in order to avoid being confronted with failures at an early stage due to exaggerated expectations regarding the extent of weight reduction. A further aim of psychotherapeutic interventions is to achieve a structured but flexibly controlled eating behaviour, as it will not be possible to maintain a permanent caloric restriction. It is also important to discuss the possibility of setbacks and to identify suitable coping strategies. Group therapies have the advantage, despite their reduced options to individualise treatment, of being able to use group dynamic and interpersonal aspects, which often play a special role in the treatment of obese patients.

Specific psychotherapy for manifest mental disorders such as depression, anxiety disorders or eating disorders, which are clearly more common in obese patients who wish to be treated, should be offered in addition to obesity treatment, if only to improve the quality of life.

In addition to the treatment of anxiety disorders and depression, there is also good evidence of psychotherapeutic treatment for binge-eating disorder, which is particularly relevant in the context of obesity treatment. There is evidence of effectiveness especially for cognitive behavioural therapy and interpersonal psychotherapy. These good results can be maintained for the most part even in the longer course over 2 years. Guided self-help programmes can also be effective for the treatment of mild forms of binge-eating with still maintained self-esteem and pronounced body image disorders. On the other hand, simple weight reduction programmes based on behavioural therapy are not suitable for significantly reducing eating attacks in the context of binge-eating disorders. It should be noted that even the successful treatment of a binge-eating disorder does not lead to pronounced effects in terms of weight loss.

Overall, the direct and indirect metabolic effects of chronic stress for the aetiology of obesity are probably still underestimated. In this respect, it will be interesting to see whether psychotherapeutic interventions aimed at stress reduction will be a fixed component of obesity-specific therapeutic procedures in the future. Furthermore, given the character of obesity as a chronic disease with a high tendency to relapse ("the weight returns when the therapy stops"), it could be decisive within the framework of conservative approaches to what extent it is possible to integrate psychotherapeutic elements into the lives of those affected in the long term.

2.5 Drug Therapy

U. Elbelt

The introduction of further drugs for the treatment of obesity is expected in the future. Currently, the lipase inhibitor orlistat and the incretin analogue liraglutide are available for the drug therapy of obesity. The approval of the selective endocannabinoid (CB1) receptor antagonist rimonabant (increased risk for depression, anxiety disorders and suicidal thoughts) and the selective serotonin and norepinephrine reuptake inhibitor sibutramine (increased risk of cardiovascular events) has been withdrawn.

2.5.1 Orlistat

Orlistat is administered in a dosage of maximum 120 mg three times daily with main meals. As a side effect of this lipase inhibitor, gastrointestinal symptoms such as meteorism, increased urge to defecate and soft stools up to diarrhoea can occur due to insufficient fat digestion. Furthermore, a reduced absorption of fat-soluble vitamins may occur. In a placebo-controlled study over a period of 4 years, weight loss under intensive lifestyle intervention and administration of placebo was 6.2 kg after 1 year and 3.0 kg after 4 years. Under therapy with orlistat and lifestyle intervention, weight loss was higher with 10.6 kg after 1 year and 5.8 kg after 4 years (Togerson et al. 2004). Orlistat has been approved for over-the-counter use at a dosage of 60 mg.

2.5.2 Liraglutide

Another effective drug is the incretin analogue liraglutide, which is already approved for diabetes therapy. In a study published in 2009, liraglutide was also used for the mdical treatment of obesity in 564 participants aged 18–65 years with a BMI between 30 and 40 kg/m^2 (Astrup et al. 2009). The participants had neither diabetes mellitus nor impaired glucose tolerance. In addition to a diet with a daily energy deficit of approximately 500 kcal and the requirement to increase physical exercise, the participants in this multi-centre, randomised, double-blind study received placebo, orlistat (120 mg three times daily) or liraglutide in ascending doses of 1.2 to a maximum of 3.0 mg/day. After 20 weeks, the average weight loss of the participants was 2.8 kg on placebo, 4.1 kg on orlistat therapy and 7.2 kg on liraglutide therapy at the maximum dosage. As a side effect, nausea was reported in about half of the paticipants receiving liraglutide at the maximum dosage, with the proportion of participants reporting nausea decreasing significantly over time.

In March 2015, liraglutide was approved in the European Union by the European Medicines Agency (EMA). This was followed in April 2016 by the market launch of liraglutide for the treatment of obesity.

Also in March 2015, the EMA approved a naltrexone/bupropion combination product in the European Union.

2.5.3 Metformin

The use of the oral antidiabetic metformin can also be considered in the context of off-label use. The recommendation of therapy with metformin in off-label use is derived from the experience with metformin therapy for diabetes prevention, the use of metformin for diabetes treatment and the administration of metformin in women with polycystic ovarian syndrome. In the A Diabetes Outcome Progression Trail (ADOPT) (Kahn et al. 2006), 4360 patients with newly diagnosed diabetes mellitus type 2 were randomised to monotherapy with rosiglitazone, metformin or glibenclamide and observed for a median follow-up of 4 years. While monotherapy with glibenclamide and rosiglitazone resulted in a weight gain of 1.6 kg and 4.8 kg, respectively, participants on monotherapy with metformin were able to reduce their weight by 2.9 kg on average. Own experience with metformin in off-label use for weight reduction in patients with impaired glucose tolerance or still maintained blood glucose control and insulin resistance in combination with a diet that largely avoids foods with a high glycemic index has shown very good results in selected patients. Well-documented patient education and careful attention to contraindications (especially kidney dysfunction with a creatinine clearance <60 ml/min) are prerequisites for off-label use.

Practical Tip

It should be noted that all three drugs described here cannot be prescribed at the expense of the statutory health insurance companies.

The question remains unanswered as to the period of time over which drug therapy should be carried out, as the available studies cover maximum periods of 4 years.

2.6 Multimodal Therapy Programmes

T. Hofmann

Multimodal therapy programmes combine the above-mentioned principles of nutrition, physical exercise and behaviour therapy in a coordinated treatment approach and are usually carried out in groups. The advantage of these combined programmes is that they are expected to be more successful than the application of single components. According to the current S3 guideline for "Prevention and therapy of obesity", programmes should be offered from a BMI of 30 kg/m^2 or—in case of secondary diseases—from a BMI of 25 kg/m^2. In each case therapy goals should be based on taking into account the individual

situation of the patient. The primary goal of weight loss treatment is to reduce body weight in the long term in order to avoid or improve obesity-related comorbidities and secondary diseases and to reduce the risk of premature mortality, incapacity to work or retirement. The sustained success of the therapy will depend largely on the patient's ability to achieve improved self-regulation. The psychosocial factors that have been identified in a meta-analysis and that have been shown to be favourable or unfavourable for sustained weight control are summarised below.

Factors Associated with Sustained Weight Control After Weight Loss (Elfhag and Rössner 2005)
- Reaching a weight target
- High initial weight loss
- Physically active lifestyle
- Regular meal rhythm
- Regular breakfast
- Less fatty food, more "healthy food"
- Less frequent consumption of snacks
- Flexibly controlled eating behaviour
- (Documented) self-monitoring
- Favourable coping strategies
- Ability to deal with craving for food (craving)
- Self-efficacy
- Autonomy
- "Healthy Narcissism"
- Confidence in your own abilities as motivation for weight loss
- Stable environment
- Ability to enter into close relationships

Factors Associated with Weight Gain Following Weight Reduction (Elfhag and Rössner 2005)
- Attribution of medical factors as the cause of obesity
- Perception of obstacles to weight-reducing behaviour
- Weight fluctuations in the history ("weight cycling")
- Inactive, sedentary lifestyle

2

- Uncontrolled, disturbed eating behaviour
- Increased feelings of hunger
- Hunger pangs
- Eating as a way of dealing with negative emotions and stress
- Psychosocial burdens
- Lack of social support
- Passive handling of problems
- Unfavourable coping strategies
- Lack of self-confidence
- Presence of psychopathological conditions
- Medical reasons or urging of other persons as motivation for weight reduction
- Dichotomous thinking

The available evaluated programmes aim at different target groups with varying degrees of obesity. Clinically significant weight reduction is usually achieved with programme lasting approximately 1 year. However, a considerable percentage of participants drops out of these programmes. Internet- and telephone-based approaches that allow for better integration into the everyday life of the participants can also achieve relevant effects. Weight loss with these programmes is usually less pronounced than in programmes based on face-to-face interventions. As the initial effects of conservative weight loss programmes on body weight can generally not be maintained over a longer period of time, or only to a limited extent, and as overall mortality cannot be significantly reduced even with longer-term interventions, a reorientation with regard to the primary therapeutic goals should be considered in addition to further improvement of the programmes. Lifestyle intervention programmes are able to achieve improvements, particularly in the physical quality of life, or to delay deterioration and reduce the incidence of depressive disorders, with the patients with the lowest quality of life appearing to benefit most. These aspects are highly relevant for the treatment of obese people. In this respect, multimodal therapy programmes should also be important components in the treatment of obesity, regardless of the indication for bariatric surgery. Prior to bariatric surgery, they can also make a significant contribution to structuring everyday life and eating behaviour or counteract unfavourable social withdrawal tendencies. In addition, the ability to regulate emotions as well as the emotional functionality of eating can be addressed even before the anatomical and metabolic changes of the operations with their requirements for a change in eating behaviour.

References

Astrup A, Rössner S, Van Gaal L et al (2009) Effects of liraglutide in the treatment of obesity: a randomised, double-blind, placebo-controlled study. Lancet 374:1606–1616

Dansinger ML, Gleason JA, Griffith JL, Selker HP, Schaefer EJ (2005) Comparison of the Atkins, Ornish, Weight watchers, and zone diets for weight loss and heart disease risk reduction: a randomized trial. JAMA 293:43–53

Deutsche Adipositas-Gesellschaft, Deutsche Diabetes Gesellschaft, Deutsche Gesellschaft für Ernährung, deutsche Gesellschaft für Ernährungsmedizin (2014) Interdisziplinäre Leitlinie der Qualität S3 zur "Prävention und Therapie der Adipositas". AWMF-Register Nr. 050/001. Klasse: S3. Version 2.0. http://www.adipositas-gesellschaft.de/fileadmin/PDF/Leitlinien/S3_Adipositas_Praevention_Therapie_2014.pdf. (25. April 2016)

Deutsche Gesellschaft für Ernährung (DGE) (2009) DGE Beratungs-standards. Graphoprint Verlag Ruth Schlotter, Koblenz

Deutsche Gesellschaft für Ernährung (DGE), Österreichische Gesellschaft für Ernährung (ÖGE), Schweizerische Gesellschaft für Ernährungsforschung (SGE), Schweizerische Vereinigung für Ernährung (2008) Referenzwerte für die Nährstoffzufuhr. Neuer Umschau Buchverlag, Neustadt/Weinstraße

Elfhag K, Rössner S (2005) Who succeeds in maintaining weight loss? A conceptual review of factors associated with weight loss maintenance and weight regain. Obes Rev 6:67–85

Franz MJ, van Wormer JJ, Crain AL et al (2007) Weight-loss outcomes: a systematic review and meta-analysis of weight-loss clinical trials with a minimum 1-year follow-up. J Am Diet Assoc 107:1755–1767

Kahn SE, Haffner SM, Heise MA et al (2006) Glycemic durability of rosiglitazone, metformin, or glyburide monotherapy. N Engl J Med 355:2427–2443

Sacks FM, Bray GA, Carey VJ et al (2009) Comparison of weight-loss diets with different compositions of fat, protein, and carbohydrates. N Engl J Med 360:859–873

Shai I, Schwarzfuchs D, Henkin Y et al (2008) Weight loss with a low-carbohydrate, Mediterranean, or low-fat diet. N Engl J Med 359:229–241

Thomas JG, Bond DS, Phelan S, Hill JO, Wing RR (2014) Weight-loss maintenance for 10 years in the National Weight Control Registry. Am J Prev Med 46:17–23

Torgerson JS, Hauptman J, Boldrin MN, Sjöström L (2004) XENical in the prevention of diabetes in obese subjects (XENDOS) study: a randomized study of orlistat as an adjunct to lifestyle changes for the prevention of type 2 diabetes in obese patients. Diabetes Care 27:155–161

Wing RR, Hill JO (2001) Successful weight loss maintenance. Annu Rev Nutr 21:323–341

Further Readings

Haslam DW, James WPT (2005) Obesity Lancet 366:1197–1209

Hauner H (2015) Ernährungsmedizinische Konzepte bei Adipositas. Internist 56:137–142

Iacovino JM, Gredysa DM, Altman M, Wilfley DE (2012) Psychological treatments for binge eating disorder. Curr Psychiatry Rep 14:432–446

Kushner RF, Elbelt U, Scholze JE (2012) Diagnostik und Management der Adipositas. In: Longo DL, Fauci AS, Kaspar DL, et al. (Hrsg.) Harrisons Innere Medizin. ABW Wissenschaftsverlag, Berlin, S673–681

Kushner RF, Ryan DH (2014) Assessment and lifestyle management of patients with obesity: clinical recommendations from systematic reviews. JAMA 312:943–952

Shaw K, O'Rourke P, Del Mar C, Kenardy J (2005) Psychological interventions for overweight or obesity. Cochrane Database Syst Rev 18:2

Thompson D, Karpe F, Lafontan M, Frayn K (2012) Physical activity and exercise in the regulation of human adipose tissue physiology. Physiol Rev 92:157–191

Surgical Therapy of Obesity

J. Ordemann and A. Stengel

Contents

© Springer-Verlag GmbH Germany, part of Springer Nature 2022
J. Ordemann, U. Elbelt (eds.), *Obesity and Metabolic Surgery*,
https://doi.org/10.1007/978-3-662-63227-7_3

3

3.1 Frequency of Obesity Surgery

J. Ordemann

The surgical treatment of severe obesity has proven to be very effective and sustainable. Diet and exercise therapy ("lifestyle intervention") as well as drug therapy usually do not show sufficient or lasting effects. In contrast, bariatric surgery leads to long-term weight reduction and also to an improvement in obesity-related diseases. Since several prospective, randomized studies and meta-analyses have shown superiority over conservative therapy, the evidence is well established. Weight-loss surgery has established itself in the treatment concept of obese patients as well as in the therapy of metabolic secondary diseases. The introduction of the laparoscopic surgical technique has significantly reduced morbidity and mortality.

For the reasons mentioned above and due to the increasing number of patients with high-grade obesity, bariatric surgery has become one of the most common surgical procedures within visceral surgery. More than 300,000 operations are performed worldwide every year. In relation to population size, the most frequent operations are performed in Sweden, Belgium and the USA, among others. In comparison, surgical interventions are rare in Germany with an operation frequency of 11 operations per 100,000 inhabitants (◨ Fig. 3.1). Germany is underserved in regard to the frequency of bariatric interventions. Less than 1% of those patients with high obesity for whom surgery is indicated according to the S3 guidelines of the medical societies actually receive bariatric surgery in Germany.

A major reason for this low number of operations is the approval practice of the health insurance companies in Germany. The lengthy and bureaucratic application procedure is very stressful for many of those affected, and in most cases indicated operations are delayed, which in individual cases has considerable health consequences. For doctors experienced in obesity therapy, the recommendations of the Medical Service of the Health Insurance Funds (MDK) are in most cases not comprehensive. In addition, there are regional differences in care within Germany. They illustrate the sometimes incomprehensive assessment practice of the regional MDKs (◨ Fig. 3.2).

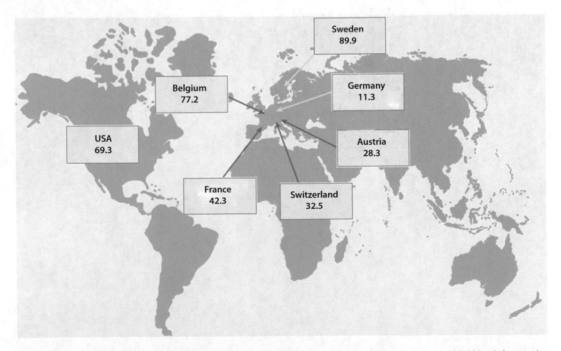

◨ **Fig. 3.1** Obesity surgery in international comparison. Number of annual operations per 100,000 adult population. (From Weiner 2015, with kind permission)

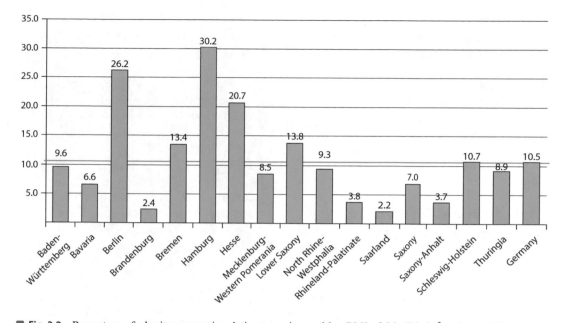

▣ Fig. 3.2 Percentage of obesity surgery in relation to patients with a BMI of 35–40 kg/m² and type 2 diabetes or BMI > 40 kg/m². (Adapted from Hüttl et al. 2015, with kind permission)

With increasing knowledge about the effectiveness of bariatric surgery and in particular about improving blood glucose control in type 2 diabetes, a significant increase in the frequency of operations is also expected in Germany. Taking into account the massively increasing number of severely obese patients and the scientific evidence of the very good effectiveness of surgical therapy, health insurance companies will no longer be able to evade this responsibility in the future. However, it is likely that only the decisions of the social courts will confirm the rights of patients and thus enable them to have adequate access to the necessary surgical therapy.

Therefore, the number of surgical interventions in Germany will reach the European average in the future, rising to 20,000–30,000 interventions per year.

3.2 Therapeutic Goals and Evaluation Criteria

In addition to weight reduction, the goals of an obesity surgery are the improvement of obesity-associated diseases and an increase in the quality of life. Furthermore, weight-loss surgery leads to a reduction in new diseases such as type 2 diabetes and arterial hypertension and therefore serves as a preventive measure.

Usually, bariatric therapy is based on a normal weight, which is calculated from the body height (in cm) minus 100 kg. Excess weight is the weight that exceeds the normal weight. If this excess weight is reduced by bariatric surgery, this reduction is known as "excess weight loss" (EWL). A reduction in excess weight of at least 50% (EWL 50%) is defined as a therapeutic success in bariatric surgery. However, the sole reference to this parameter is not sufficient to assess the success of treatment, as positive influences of bariatric surgery on comorbidity and quality of life are not taken into account.

In view of numerous large studies, it can be assumed that after obesity surgery, an EWL of over 60% as well as a (temporary) remission of type 2 diabetes in 77%, arterial hypertension in 62% and sleep apnea syndrome in over 80% of cases can be achieved. These data published in 2004 by Buchwald et al. (2004) were confirmed in further meta-analyses of both short and long-term observations.

3

> **Conclusion**
> Obesity surgery has the following goals:
> - Long-term and sustainable weight reduction of at least 50% of overweight
> - Improvement or remission of obesity-related secondary diseases
> - Improving the quality of life
> - Prevention of secondary diseases
> - Reducing mortality due to obesity
> - Reducing obesity-related expenses

3.3 Indications for Surgical Treatment of Obesity

J. Ordemann

The indications for bariatric surgery are still not conclusively clarified and are subject to constant change. Currently valid are the S3 guideline "Surgery of Obesity", published 2010 by the German Society for General and Visceral Surgery, and the interdisciplinary S3 guideline "Prevention and Therapy of Obesity", published 2014 by the German Obesity Society, the German Diabetes Society, the German Nutrition Society and the German Society for Nutritional Medicine. Future guidelines will probably include an expansion of the indications for surgical therapy of obesity and its secondary diseases.

According to the current guidelines, an obesity surgical intervention can be carried out from a BMI > 40 kg/m^2 (grade III obesity) or between >35 and <40 kg/m^2 (grade II obesity) and the additional presence of considerable comorbidities, provided that conservative treatment options have been exhausted. In individual cases, obesity surgery can also be performed on patients with type 2 diabetes and grade I obesity (BMI > 30 and <35 kg/m^2). It should be noted that an obesity surgery can also be performed without preoperative conservative therapy, if this is without any prospect of success or if the patient's state of health does not allow postponement of the operation.

> **Indications for Bariatric Surgery**
> Surgical indication is given with:
> - BMI > 40 kg/m^2 or
> - BMI > 35 kg/m^2 with significant comorbidities and unsuccessful multimodal conservative therapy over 6 months within the last 2 years
>
> Surgical treatment of obesity can, however, also be carried out without preoperative conservative therapy if conservative therapy has no prospect of success or the patient's state of health does not permit postponement of the operation. This applies to the following cases:
> - BMI > 50 kg/m^2
> - Particular severity of concomitant and secondary diseases of obesity
> - Psychosocial circumstances that do not hold out the prospect of a successful lifestyle change

3.4 Obesity Surgical Procedures

J. Ordemann

The spectrum and indication of surgical interventions are subject to constant change. In the 1950s the first operations were being performed to reduce the overweight of severely obese patients. In the 1960s, Edward Mason developed the gastric bypass. In the mid-1970s Nicola Scopinaro developed the biliopancreatic bypass. In 1994 the first gastric bypass operation was performed laparoscopically. At the same time the implantation of the gastric band was established. These continuous changes are divided into three phases in the publication "Changing Trends in Bariatric Surgery" by Lo Menzo et al. (2015): the pioneering phase in the 1950s and 1960s, the laparoscopic phase in the 1990s and the metabolic phase at present. In Germany, there has also been a shift in the different surgical procedures over the past decades. While in

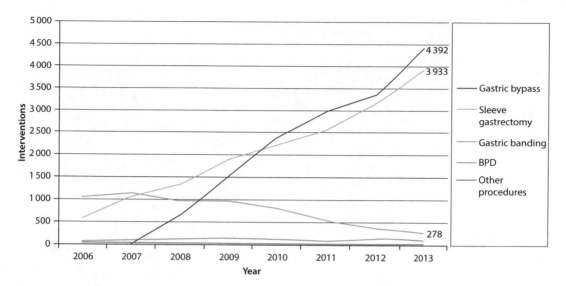

Fig. 3.3 Process selection in Germany. Development of bariatric interventions between 2006 and 2013. (Adapted from Hüttl et al. 2015, with kind permission)

the 1990s the gastric band implantation was most often performed, today the laparoscopic sleeve gastrectomy and the laparoscopic gastric bypass are the most frequently performed procedures (■ Fig. 3.3).

3.4.1 Laparoscopic Adjustable Gastric Banding

Before 2007, the implantation of an adjustable gastric band (■ Fig. 3.4) was one of the most frequent obesity surgery procedures in Germany. In the meantime, this operation is rarely performed and accounts for fewer than 3% of all interventions. In gastric band implantation, food restriction is achieved by forming a small stomach pouch. The laparoscopic placement of the adjustable silicone band is performed slightly below the entrance to the stomach. The degree of restriction can be adjusted with the controllable gastric bands via a port system.

However, it is problematic that energy-rich liquid food can be absorbed unhindered. Often it is therefore not possible to achieve sufficient weight reduction. Laparoscopic implantation is described in detail in ▶ Chap. 8.

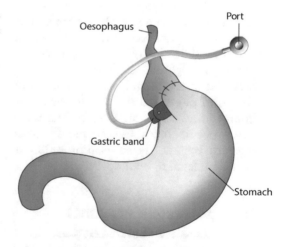

Fig. 3.4 Laparoscopic gastric band

3.4.2 Laparoscopic Sleeve Gastrectomy

Sleeve gastrectomy (■ Fig. 3.5) was originally used for biliopancreatic diversion with duodenal switch. In the meantime, sleeve gastrectomy is performed as a stand-alone procedure and is the most frequently performed bariatric procedure in Germany. In laparoscopic sleeve gastrectomy, a large part of the stomach is resected, leaving a tubular residual stomach.

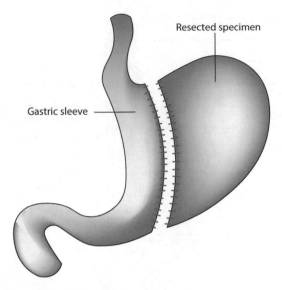

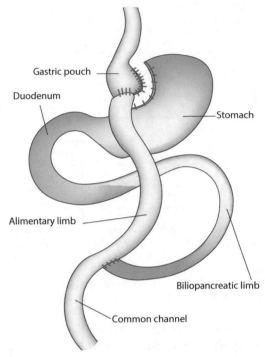

◘ **Fig. 3.5** Sleeve gastrectomy

The working principle consists on the one hand of food restriction, on the other hand of altered humoral peptide hormone levels, which lead to a modification of hunger and satiety. The average weight reduction is 60–70% after 2 years. The intervention is not reversible, but has the advantages that the gastric passage is maintained and a lack of vitamins and trace elements occurs much less frequently than with gastric bypass. The surgical procedure is described in detail in ▶ Chap. 9.

◘ **Fig. 3.6** Proximal gastric bypass

pouch anastomosis and approximately 50 cm aborally from the Treitz's arch.

The average weight loss of patients is about 60–75% of the excess weight after 2 years. A detailed description of the operation can be found in ▶ Chap. 10.

3.4.3 **Laparoscopic Proximal Roux-en-Y Gastric Bypass**

Roux-en-Y- gastric bypass (◘ Fig. 3.6) is still considered the gold standard in obesity and metabolic surgery. The gastric bypass combines restriction and malabsorption and leads to altered regulation of hunger and satiety due to modified hormonal and neuronal signals. When a gastric bypass is performed, a small stomach pouch is formed. This is anastomosed with a jejunum loop switched off after Roux-Y. A large part of the stomach, the duodenum and part of the jejunum are thus separated from the food passage. The jejunojejunal anastomosis is performed at approximately 120–150 cm aborally from the

3.4.4 **One-Anastomosis Laparoscopic Bypass**

The omega-loop gastric bypass (◘ Fig. 3.7) was developed in the USA in 1997. Today, this operation is also being performed more and more frequently in Germany. Similar to the gastric bypass, the food passage through the duodenum is switched off. The reduction in the size of the stomach is similar to a gastric bypass, but there is no resection of parts of the stomach and the Aa. and Vv. gastricae breves are preserved. The reduced stomach is anastomosed with a small intestinal loop. The biliary loop measures about 200 cm aborally from the Treitz's arch.

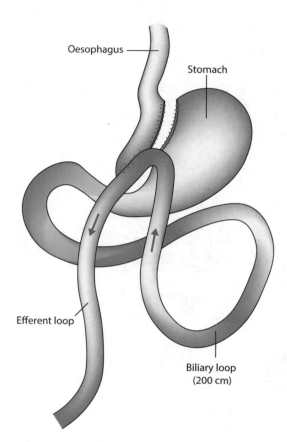

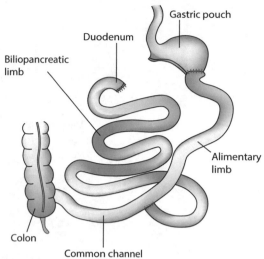

□ Fig. 3.8   Biliopancreatic diversion by Scopinaro

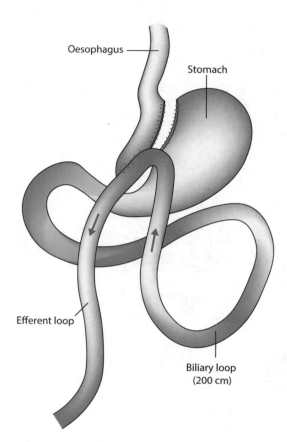

□ Fig. 3.7   Omega-loop gastric bypass

The operation is suitable as a primary operation or as a second step after the application of a sleeve gastrectomy. A detailed description of the surgical technique is given in ▶ Chap. 11.

3.4.5   Biliopancreatic Diversion (According to Scopinaro)

The biliopancreatic diversion (BPD) according to Scopinaro (□ Fig. 3.8) is used very rarely in Germany with fewer than 1% being performed. Scopinaro developed this technique in 1979. Biliopancreatic diversion enables safe weight reduction and good remission rates of type 2 diabetes, but is associated with an unfavorable side effect profile due to malabsorption and increased perioperative complications. Duodenal exclusion and the long biliopancreatic loop in combination with the very short common channel result in complex hormonal and metabolic changes. The operation is described in detail in ▶ Chap. 12.

3.4.6   Biliopancreatic Diversion with Duodenal Switch

Biliopancreatic diversion with Duodenal Switch (BPD-DS) combines restriction (sleeve gastrectomy) with malabsorption by Roux-en-Y reconstruction with a short common channel (□ Fig. 3.9). The small intestine is largely separated from the food passage. This results in a considerable malabsorption of fats, vitamins and trace elements. As a result, there is strong weight reduction and very favourable improvements in obesity-associated secondary diseases, primarily type 2 diabetes. However, the risk of malnutrition is very high. For this reason, this operation is now performed only very rarely and in specialised clinics (▶ Chap. 13).

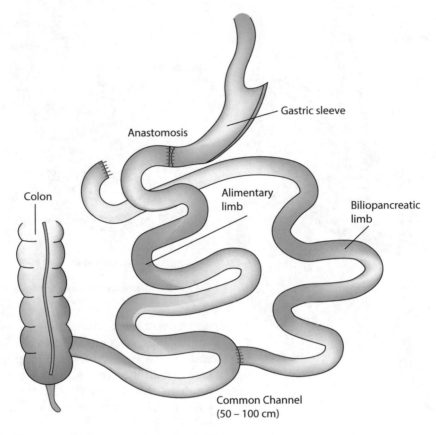

Fig. 3.9 Biliopancreatic diversion with duodenal switch

3.5 Mechanisms of Action

J. Ordemann

The significance of classically assumed mechanisms of action such as restriction and malabsorption is increasingly being questioned. Biophysiological mechanisms of action, which have a direct influence on hunger and satiety as well as food preference, seem to be much more plausible in explaining the favourable results of surgical therapy. The scientific interest is mainly focused on the effect of gastrointestinal peptide hormones. Possible further factors that have an influence on postoperative body weight regulation and metabolic secondary diseases are changes in the intestinal microbiome and shifts in the concentration of bile acids in the serum. Despite extensive clinical experience and experimental animal studies, the integration of these numerous findings

into a comprehensive understanding of the mechanisms of action of bariatric surgery is still pending.

In order to be able to provide optimal care for patients undergoing obesity surgery, the attending physicians must understand the mechanisms of action of the different surgical interventions for the digestive tract and metabolism. This understanding not only plays a significant role in the selection of a bariatric procedure, but is also indispensable for the aftercare of the patients.

Initially, obesity surgery was developed and performed to reduce the patients' food and energy intake. A reduction in the size of the stomach (restriction) and a deliberate lack of digestion (malabsorption) were the presumed "key mechanisms". Historically, obesity surgery has been divided into restrictive procedures, malabsorptive procedures and combined procedures.

Obesity Surgical Procedures

Restrictive procedures: Surgical interventions that limit the food supply. These include gastric banding and sleeve gastrectomy.

Malabsorptive procedures: Surgical interventions that limit the absorption of food components. The classic procedure is biliopancreatic diversion (BPD) according to Scopinaro.

Combined procedures: Surgical interventions using restrictive and malabsorptive mechanisms of action. Gastric bypass is a restrictive procedure with discrete malabsorptive effects. Biliopancreatic diversion with duodenal switch is also a classic combination procedure.

Basically, restriction and malabsorption are important mechanisms of action in reducing body weight. Their importance in the attempt to explain the phenomenon decreases with increasing knowledge of the biophysiological changes. However, these mechanisms of action still play an important role in the aftercare of patients and in the therapy of complications after obesity surgery. ▶ Section 3.5.1 discusses this in more detail.

Gastrointestinal peptide hormones are of major importance for the explanation of the mechanisms of action. Anatomical changes in the digestive tract due to partial exclusion of the stomach and duodenum during gastric bypass or the resection of a large part of the stomach during sleeve gastrectomy lead to a modified secretion of numerous gastrointestinal hormones. Glucagon-like peptide 1, peptide YY and ghrelin are only a few representatives of these hormones, whose effect is demonstrably increased or weakened by the surgical intervention. These changes are explained in detail in ▶ Sect. 3.5.2.

Further interesting results are obtained by observing the intestinal flora. The microbiome of the intestine seems to be modified by bariatric interventions to such an extent that this could have a direct influence on the

results of the surgical interventions. This is discussed in ▶ Sect. 3.5.3. Fluctuations in the concentration of bile acids in the intestine and serum after bariatric surgery also provide new explanations for the mechanisms of action of bariatric surgery. This is reported on in ▶ Sect. 3.5.4.

In addition to changes in the gut-brain axis, the bacterial composition of the intestinal flora and the concentration of bile acids, other mechanisms probably play a role in weight regulation. An increase in the basal metabolic rate after obesity surgery, altered vagal information transmission and changes in hepatic metabolic processes are regarded as possible triggers that could have a direct and indirect influence on body weight regulation.

The considerations of a hypothetical "setpoint" of weight regulation, which keeps body weight within narrow limits by "individual imprinting" and external environmental factors are advanced. Due to the surgical changes with their effects on, among other things, the gut-brain axis and the intestinal microbiome, this "setpoint" will probably be strongly down-regulated, so that an initial weight loss as well as long-term weight control will be possible. "Dieting" is no longer perceived as torture, but is largely perceived as a normal condition.

3.5.1 Restriction and Malabsorption

The obesity surgery was developed under the assumption of the mechanisms of action restriction and malabsorption. These exclusive explanatory approaches are now outdated, as there is increasing knowledge about changes in hormonal regulation, intestinal flora and bile acids after bariatric surgery, which have a strong influence on hunger and satiety regulation.

Restriction

Restriction means a reduction in the size of the gastric reservoir and a narrowing of the passage to the rest of the digestive tract. The result is a build-up of solid food and a premature feeling of satiety. The principle of restriction alone occurs with the gastric band. The stomach is divided into a small fore-stomach and the rest of the stomach by a gastric band. The band creates a constriction which is difficult for solid food to pass through, but easy for liquid food. The degree of restriction can be adjusted by filling the gastric band with liquid. There are no effects in the sense of malabsorption. Also changes of the intestinal-brain-axis are not achieved directly, so that a change of the "setpoint" of weight regulation is probably not possible.

The sleeve gastrectomy is also one of the restrictive procedures. Initially, sleeve gastrectomy was used as the first step before biliopancreatic diversion with duodenal switch in particularly obese patients in order to achieve weight reduction initially via a restrictive mechanism. It quickly became clear, however, that considerable weight reduction could be achieved with sleeve gastrectomy alone. Irrespective of the restrictive effect, the application of a gastric sleeve leads to changes in the secretion of gastrointestinal peptide hormones. The pure restriction seems to be of minor importance for the weight regulating effect. There is no binding recommendation for the degree of restriction in the gastric sleeve (width of the calibration tube).

A restrictive active component is also present in gastric bypass. The restriction is achieved both by the pouch size and the diameter of the gastrojejunostomy, so that the passage of solid food components into the small intestine is hindered. Liquid food can easily pass through the narrow passage as in the gastric band. The smaller the pouch and the tighter the anastomosis, the more pronounced the weight reduction. However, whether this is explained by the mechanism of action of the restriction is still a matter of controversy. It must be assumed that the anastomosis can widen in the long-term course. In the case of "poor" eating habits the extension of both the pouch and the alimentary loop is possible. In this case a renewed increase in weight will regularly occur. Therefore some surgeons advocate additional restriction by means of a band around the gastric pouch ("banded" gastric bypass). However, the increased rate of complications caused by the band itself must be taken into account. Another possibility to increase the restriction and also to prevent dilatation of the pouch is the application of a ring-enforced gastric bypass (Fobi technique).

Malabsorption

The physiological principle of malabsorption is achieved by a delayed binding of food with digestive secretions (pancreatic and bile secretions). The aim is to reduce the absorption of fats and carbohydrates. A classic malabsorptive procedure is the biliopancreatic diversion according to Scopinaro. The extent of malabsorption is defined by the length of the common channel, which can be between 50 and 125 cm long. This procedure leads to the greatest weight reduction compared to all other obesity surgical procedures because of its considerable malabsorption. The malabsorption is associated with a strong loss of macro- and micronutrients. Depending on the extent of malabsorption, fatty stools and diarrhoea can occur. Especially in the case of biliopancreatic diversion, the malabsorptive effect can be so pronounced that the long-term consequences can be considerable. Consistent substitution and lifelong aftercare with regular blood tests are essential. Otherwise, clinical complications are unavoidable.

The gastric bypass combines a very mild malabsorption with the restriction. The difficult resorption of macronutrients during the proximal gastric bypass is usually sufficiently compensated by the residual small intestine. The reduced absorption of micronutrients caused by the exclusion of duodenum and part of the jejunum must be taken into account. Secondary hyperparathyroidism is a typical consequence of limited calcium absorption and hypovitaminosis D_3.

A more complex situation exists with distal gastric bypass and also with omega bypass. These operations usually lead to an increased weight reduction compared to the proximal gastric bypass. The shorter common channel in longer biliopancreatic slings (omega bypass 200 cm) leads to a more pronounced restriction of fat resorption.

3.5.2   Effects of Bariatric Surgery on the Regulation of Hunger and Satiety

A. Stengel

Contrary to the original assumption of pure restriction or malabsorption as underlying factors for the significant weight loss and metabolic changes after bariatric surgery, a significant involvement of gastrointestinal peptide hormones is increasingly assumed. While after conservative weight loss attempts compensatory changes of these hormones can often be observed, which counteract further weight loss, a different picture emerges after bariatric surgery. Postoperatively, a reduction of the (orexigenic) hormone ghrelin, which leads to hunger, as well as an increase in various (anorexigenic) hormones, which lead to satiation, is observed. These altered regulatory mechanisms are described below.

Ghrelin

Measurements have shown that ghrelin levels decrease after bariatric surgery and increase after diet-induced weight loss. Thus, gastric bypass surgery led to a significant reduction in circulating ghrelin concentrations; the meal-dependent or diurnal modulation of ghrelin can no longer be observed postoperatively. This reduction is explained by the exclusion of the gastric passage or by resection of the gastric fundus. The activation of the ghrelin cells localized in the fundus is thus reduced. This observation is supported by histological studies which have shown a lower postoperative ghrelin mRNA expression in the fundus.

However, some studies have described that the ghrelin concentration does not decrease after gastric bypass surgery. One explanation could be the functional (residual) activity, which possibly correlates with the size of the gastric pouch and, in the case of a large pouch, also includes parts of the fundus, so that there may still be contact between the chyme and the fundus.

As expected, the ghrelin values decrease strongly after a sleeve gastrectomy, since the fundus is largely resected in this surgical procedure. In addition to the (functional) integrity of the fundus, the vagus nerve seems to be important for ghrelin stimulation; thus, the decrease of ghrelin could be associated with an intraoperative effect or damage of the gastric fibers of the vagus nerve. Since ghrelin levels show a close inverse correlation with insulin sensitivity, this modulation is associated not only with a reduction in the feeling of hunger but also with an improvement in the observed glucose control. In addition, ghrelin reduction seems to play a role in the postoperatively observed improvement of cognitive functions.

However, it should be noted that the decrease in ghrelin does not alone seem to be decisive for the postoperative change in hunger and satiety regulation, as ghrelin levels in patients with good weight loss do not differ from those with an insufficient weight response. It is also not possible to predict weight loss based on preoperative ghrelin levels or postoperative changes in this hormone.

Nesfatin-1

In rats, gastric bypass led to an increase in circulating NUCB2/nesfatin-1 levels, which could contribute to improved glucose tolerance and body weight loss. Interestingly, this increase in plasma NUCB2/nesfatin-1 levels was not observed in rats after sleeve gastrectomy, so gastric bypass has a more beneficial effect on the regulation of NUCB2/nesfatin-1. It is still unclear whether an altered vagal regulation plays a role here. In a pilot study in humans, however, both gastric bypass surgery and sleeve gastrectomy led to a reduction in circulating NUCB2/nesfatin-1 levels in plasma. This result should first be replicated in larger studies and, if confirmed, investigated for other influencing variables.

Cholecystokinin

Cholecystokinin levels also increase after bariatric surgery, with sleeve gastrectomy leading to significantly higher postprandial cholecystokinin concentrations than gastric bypass surgery. This postoperative increase could be caused by an increased number of cholecystokinin-producing cells in the small intestine - resulting in increased saturation and thus a reduction in body weight.

Pancreatic Polypeptide

The changes in the pancreatic polypeptide are not clear. While a reduction was observed in one study after a gastric bypass, the levels were elevated after sleeve gastrectomy. However, the pancreatic polypeptide levels do not seem to have a significant influence on postoperative saturation regulation, as the hormone levels did not differ between patients with favourable and unfavourable responses.

Peptide YY

The postprandial peptide YY is increased after bariatric surgery but not after diet-induced weight loss. This could contribute to an increased satiety signal and reduced feeling of hunger. It should be noted that in patients who responded poorly to surgery, the postprandial response of peptide YY was less pronounced than in patients who responded successfully. These results support the assumption of a regulatory role of peptide YY in postoperative satiety regulation as well as weight loss.

In comparison to sleeve gastrectomy, the increase in peptide YY is more pronounced after a gastric bypass. Interestingly, a further increase of peptide YY was observed after additional fundus resection in the process of a gastric bypass operation. After this operation, an increase in peptide YY-producing L-cells was observed in the small intestine. The changes in peptide YY were detectable immediately after the operation and well before the weight-reducing effect of the operation. This could indicate hormonal and/or nervous influences.

Glucagon-Like Peptide 1

Numerous studies have shown that gastric bypass surgery leads to a pronounced increase in postprandial glucagon-like peptide 1 (GLP-1) secretion. In patients with diabetes type 2 a significant reduction in the release of meal-dependent GLP-1 secretion can once again detected. Furthermore, the combination of gastric bypass surgery and fundus resection led to an additional stimulation of postpran-dial GLP-1 secretion. This observation could also be related to an altered vagal signal transmission. A modulation of GLP-1 secretion can also be observed after gastrectomy. The effect occurs independently of weight loss very early (within days) after surgery and seems to be long-lasting. In the small intestine an increase of GLP-1-producing L-cells can be observed. Interestingly, a stimulation of the expression and release of GLP-1 by bile acids could be shown in vitro, so that the postoperative observed increase of circulating bile acids could also have a favourable effect. The modulation of GLP-1 signaling seems to take place mainly at the ligand level, since the receptor expression in the pancreatic endocrine islets was not changed postoperatively.

The postoperative increased release of GLP-1 led to an increase in insulin secretion and the changes in glucagon release led to an increase in insulin sensitivity. This leads to an overall improvement/restoration of glucose control. However, these changes can also be excessive and result in postprandial hypoglycaemia (▶ Sect. 14.8.1). This can be corrected by the application of a GLP-1 receptor antagonist.

Leptin

Since leptin correlates closely with fat mass, a significant reduction (75%) in circulating leptin levels is observed after bariatric surgery. In this context, the fat cell volume seems to be of particular importance, but the fat mass or the body mass index is not as important. For this reason, leptin levels also decrease disproportionately compared to changes in the body mass index. This change can be observed after gastric bypass as well as after sleeve gastrectomy. The decrease of leptin is visible a few weeks after the operation. In addition to a reduction of leptin due to decreased production, a decrease in free leptin due to postoperative upregulation of soluble leptin receptor may also play a role. Overall, in addition to direct effects on food intake and body weight, these changes may also affect cognitive skills, as lower postoperative leptin levels are associated with improved attention and computer test performance.

Insulin

In the animal model (adult, normal-weight mini-pigs) an increased postoperative insulin release after gastric bypass surgery was observed. It is probably related to an increase in beta cell mass, the number of endocrine islets and the number of extrainsular beta cells. This increased insulin secretion was not observed in humans compared to controls, but insulin secretion is more pronounced compared to the preoperative state; postprandial saturation, which was reported to be increased, may also be a consequence. However, it should be noted that although the preoperatively disturbed beta cell function is improved, normal function cannot be achieved postoperatively. These effects can be observed after gastric bypass as well as after sleeve gastrectomy; a further increase of the postprandial insulin response could be achieved by an additional fundus resection.

Glucagon

In humans, post operation glucagon fasting levels are not changed compared to the preoperative situation. In the longer term, there is a postprandial decrease in glucagon levels after gastric bypass surgery.

Conclusion

The above section makes it clear that hormonal changes play a significant role in the regulation of favorable postoperative effects on food intake, body weight, glucose control and also other functions such as cognition. Study results that appear discrepant at first glance could be based on different surgical techniques (pouch size, vagus damage, etc.). Furthermore, it should be emphasized that no single hormone is responsible for the changes; on the contrary, the system is very pliable and allows major compensation possibilities.

3.5.3 Intestinal Flora (Microbiome)

J. Ordemann

An increasing number of studies prove that human health is directly linked to the microbiome of the intestine. Among the numerous physiological functions of the intestinal flora, food utilization and the influence of energy metabolism are of great importance.

On the other hand, there are pathophysiological functions of the intestinal microbiome with direct influence on, among other things, chronic inflammatory intestinal diseases, allergies and obesity. The composition of modern food seems to influence the intestinal microbiome and change the spectrum of germ composition. It is possible that the microbiome has a greater influence on the development of obesity than the genetic predisposition of the patients concerned. The germ spectrum, which is altered by external factors, may modulate specific signalling pathways for hunger and satiety, the utilization of nutrients and the control of energy balance. Clinical studies have shown that the microbiome of obese people differs from that of people of normal weight in terms of the composition of germs.

Animal studies have shown that the fecal transplantation of the microbiota of overweight individuals into the intestines of normal-weight, germ-free mice induces obesity. The transplantation of stool samples taken from identical twins with significantly different body weight into germ-free mice also induced a differential development of body weight in these mice. These studies suggest that "adipogenic" human microbiome is capable of increasing the body weight of obese mice.

In this respect, the question arises to what extent bariatric interventions result in a changed composition of the intestinal microbiome. A clinical pilot study from Dresden (Graessler

3

et al. 2013) showed an altered intestinal microbiome after a gastric bypass. In addition, a postoperative improvement of glucose regulation in patients with type 2 diabetes was observed. This improvement was associated with the change of the microbiome.

A pioneering study from Gothenburg (Tremaroli et al. 2015) shows that obesity surgery also leads to a long-term change in the microbiome (☐ Fig. 3.10). In this 9-year longitudinal study 21 subjects were examined. Seven patients underwent gastric bypass surgery, seven received vertical gastroplasty (VBG) and another seven did not undergo surgery and served as a control group. The microbiome of all subjects was analysed

and the energy metabolism and biochemical parameters were determined. After 9 years, the microbiome of the patients was transferred to the intestines of aseptic mice in order to establish a causal relationship between the altered microbiome of the patients who had been operated on and the weight development in the mice that received the transplants. It was shown that both surgical procedures resulted in a permanent change in the microbiome of the patients. The transplantation of the microbiome of the postoperative patients into the intestines of the germ-free mice led - with the same diet of the mice—to a lower weight gain of the mice than the transplantation of the microbiome of untreated patients.

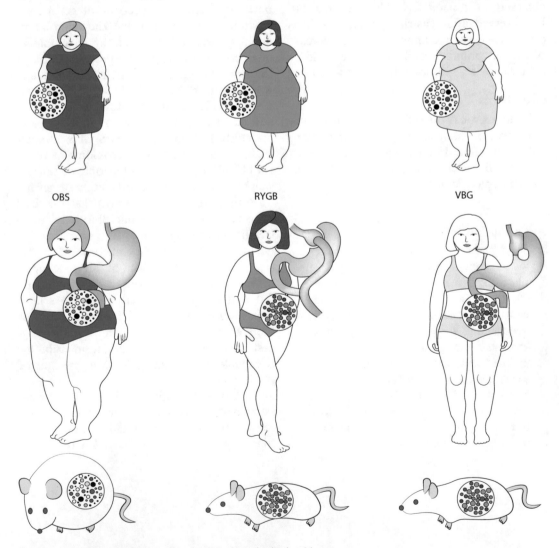

OBS   RYGB   VBG

☐ **Fig. 3.10**   Effect of obesity surgery on the intestinal microbiome

> **Conclusion**
> The study results presented not only proof of the influence of the microbiome on body weight, but also indicated the mechanism of action of obesity surgery by the alteration of the intestinal microbiome.

3.5.4 Bile Acids

Bile acids are not only necessary for fat digestion, but they are also mediators for regulatory mechanisms in the balance of energy. Physiologically, bile acids are synthesized in the liver and released into the intestinal lumen, where they serve to absorb fats and fat-soluble vitamins. In the process, they return to the bloodstream and to the liver, thus closing the enterohepatic bile acid circuit.

In animal experiments it has been shown that oral administration of bile acids leads to reduced weight gain and increased energy metabolism. It has also been shown in animal models that the bile acid level in serum increases after gastric bypass surgery. These results were confirmed in clinical studies in humans after both sleeve gastrectomy and gastric bypass surgery.

The binding to specific bile acid receptors in the cell nuclei (including farnesoid X receptor, FXR) leads to a favourable effect on hyperglycaemia and dyslipidaemia. Further receptors are located on the cell surface (e.g. G-protein Coupled Receptor TGR5). The exact molecular biological mechanisms of action are not yet well understood. In addition, a stimulation of the release of anorexic gastrointestinal peptide hormones (especially GLP-1 and PYY) from the intestinal L-cells by the bile acids is suspected.

References

3.1–3.3

Buchwald H, Avidor Y, Braunwald E et al (2004) Bariatric surgery: a systematic review and meta-analysis. JAMA 292:1724–1737

Hüttl TP, Stauch P, Wood H, Fruhmann J (2015) Bariatrische Chirurgie. Aktuelle Ernährungsmed 40:256–274

Lo Menzo E, Szomstein S, Rosenthal RJ (2015) Changing trends in bariatric surgery. Scand J Surg 104:18–23

Weiner RA (2015) Adipositas – Wann ist der Chirurg gefragt? Dtsch Med Wochenschr 140:29–33

3.4.3

Graessler J, Qin Y, Zhong H et al (2013) Metagenomic sequencing of the human gut microbiome before and after bariatric surgery in obese patients with type 2 diabetes: correlation with inflammatory and metabolic parameters. Pharmacogenomics J 13:514–522

Tremaroli V, Karlsson F, Werling M et al (2015) Roux-en-Y gastric bypass and vertical banded gastroplasty induce long-term changes on the human gut microbiome contributing to fat mass regulation. Cell Metab 22:228–238

Further Readings

3.1–3.3

Brethauer SA, Hammel JP, Schauer PR (2009) Systematic review of sleeve gastrectomy as staging and primary bariatric procedure. Surg Obes Relat Dis 5:469–475

Buchwald H, Avidor Y, Braunwald E et al (2009) Weight and type 2 diabetes after bariatric surgery: systematic review and meta-analysis. Am J Med 122:248–256

Carlsson LM, Peltonen M, Ahlin S et al (2012) Bariatric surgery and prevention of type 2 diabetes in Swedish obese subjects. N Engl J Med 367:695–704

Deutsche Adipositas-Gesellschaft, Deutsche Diabetes Gesellschaft, Deutsche Gesellschaft für Ernährung, deutsche Gesellschaft für Ernährungsmedizin (2014) Interdisziplinäre Leitlinie der Qualität S3 zur "Prävention und Therapie der Adipositas". AWMF-Register Nr. 050/001. Klasse: S3. Version 2.0. http://www.adipositas-gesellschaft.de/fileadmin/PDF/Leitlinien/S3_Adipositas_Praevention_Therapie_2014.pdf. (25. April 2016)

Deutsche Gesellschaft für Allgemein- und Viszeralchirurgie, Chirurgische Arbeitsgemeinschaft für Adipositastherapie (CAADIP), Deutsche Adipositas-Gesellschaft (DAG), Deutsche Gesellschaft für Psychosomatische Medizin und Psychotherapie, Deutsche Gesellschaft für Ernährungsmedizin (2010) S3-Leitlinie: Chirurgie der Adipositas. http://www.adipositas-gesellschaft.de/fileadmin/PDF/Leitlinien/ADIP-6-2010.pdf. (25. April 2016)

Dixon JB, O'Brien PE, Playfair J et al (2008) Adjustable gastric banding and conventional therapy for type 2 diabetes: a randomized controlled trial. JAMA 299:316–323

Fried M, Yumuk V, Oppert JM et al (2013) Interdisciplinary European guidelines on metabolic and bariatric surgery. Obes Facts 6:449–468

Hedberg J, Sundström J, Sundbom M (2014) Duodenal switch versus Roux-en-Y gastric bypass for morbid obesity: systematic review and meta-analysis of weight results, diabetes resolution and early complications in single-centre comparisons. Obes Rev 15:555–563

3

Hüttl TP, Kramer KM, Wood H (2010) Bariatrische Chirurgie—Adipositaschirurgische Verfahren und ihre Besonderheiten. Diabetologe 8:637–646

le Roux CW, Welbourn R, Werling M et al (2007) Gut hormones as mediators of appetite and weight loss after Roux-en-Y gastric bypass. Ann Surg 246:780–785

Mingrone G, Panunzi S, De Gaetano A et al (2012) Bariatric surgery versus conventional medical therapy for type 2 diabetes. N Engl J Med 366:1577–1585

Müller MK, Wildi S, Clavien PA, Weber M (2006) Chirurgische Behandlung der morbiden Adipositas. In: Siewert JR, Rothmund M, Schumpelick V (Hrsg) Praxis der Viszeralchirurgie—Gastroenterologische Chirurgie, 2. Aufl. Springer, Heidelberg, pp. S381–389

Peterli R, Steinert RE, Woelnerhansssen B et al (2012a) Metabolic and hormonal changes after laparoscopic Roux-en-Y gastric bypass and sleeve gastrectomy: a randomized, prospective trial. Obes Surg 22:740–748

Runkel N, Colombo-Benkmann M, Hüttl TP et al (2011) Bariatric surgery. Dtsch Arztebl Int 108:341–346

Schauer DP, Arterburn DE, Livingston EH et al (2015) Impact of bariatric surgery on life expectancy in severely obese patients with diabetes: a decision analysis. Ann Surg 261:914–919

Sjöström L, Narbro K, Sjöström CD et al (2007) Effect of bariatric surgery on mortality in Swedish obese subjects. N Engl J Med 357:741–752

Sjöström L, Peltonen M, Jacobson P et al (2014) Association of bariatric surgery with long-term remission of Type 2 diabetes and with microvascular and macrovascular complications. JAMA 311:2297–2304

Zhang C, Yuan Y, Qiu C, Zhang W (2014) A meta-analysis of 2 year effect after surgery: laparoscopic Roux-en-Y gastric bypass versus laparoscopic sleeve gastrectomy for morbid obesity and diabetes mellitus. Obes Surg 24:1528–1535

3.4.1

Abdeen G, le Roux CW (2016) Mechanism underlying the weight loss and complications of Roux-en-Y gastric bypass. Review. Obes Surg 26:410–421

Billeter AT, Fischer L, Wekerle AL, Senft J, Müller-Stich B (2014) malabsorption as a therapeutic approach in bariatric surgery. Viszeralmedizin 30:198–204

Bloomberg RD, Fleishman A, Nalle JE, Herron DM, Kini S (2005) Nutritional deficiencies following bariatric surgery: what have we learned? Obes Surg 15:145–154

Chakravartty S, Tassinari D, Salerno A, Giorgakis E, Rubino F (2015) What is the mechanism behind weight loss maintenance with gastric bypass? Curr Obes Rep 4:262–268

Corteville C, Fassnacht M, Bueter M (2014) Chirurgie als pluripotentes Instrument gegen eine metabolische Erkrankung. Chirurg 85:963–968

Dixon JB, Lambert EA, Lambert GW (2015) Neuroendocrine adaptations to bariatric surgery. Mol Cell Endocrinol 418:143–152

Fobi MAL, Lee H, Fleming AW (1989) The surgical technique of the banded Roux-en-Y gastric bypass. J Obes Weight Regul 8:99–102

Kaplan LM, Seeley RJ (2012) Bariatric surgery: the road ahead. The metabolic applied research strategy initiative series. Bariatric Times 9:12–13

Malinowski SS (2006) Nutritional and metabolic complications of bariatric surgery. Am J Med Sci 331:219–225

Tadross JA, le Roux CW (2009) The mechanisms of weight loss after bariatric surgery. Int J Obes 33(Suppl. 1):S28–S32

3.4.2

Borg CM, Le Roux CW, Ghatei MA et al (2006) Progressive rise in gut hormone levels after Roux-en-Y gastric bypass suggests gut adaptation and explains altered satiety. Br J Surg 93:210–215

Cummings DE, Weigle DS, Frayo RS et al (2002) Plasma ghrelin levels after diet-induced weight loss or gastric bypass surgery. N Engl J Med 346:1623–1630

Frühbeck G, Diez Caballero A, Gil MJ (2004) Fundus functionality and ghrelin concentrations after bariatric surgery. N Engl J Med 350:308–309

Karamanakos SN, Vagenas K, Kalfarentzos F, Alexandrides TK (2008) Weight loss, appetite suppression, and changes in fasting and postprandial ghrelin and peptide-YY levels after Roux-en-Y gastric bypass and sleeve gastrectomy: a prospective, double blind study. Ann Surg 247:401–407

Peterli R, Steinert RE, Woelnerhanssen B et al (2012b) Metabolic and hormonal changes after laparoscopic Roux-en-Y gastric bypass and sleeve gastrectomy: a randomized, prospective trial. Obes Surg 22:740–748

Sundbom M, Holdstock C, Engstrom BE, Karlsson FA (2007) Early changes in ghrelin following Roux-en-Y gastric bypass: influence of vagal nerve functionality? Obes Surg 17:304–310

3.4.3

Liou AP, Paziuk M, Luevano JM Jr et al (2013) Conserved shifts in the gut microbiota due to gastric bypass reduce host weight and adiposity. Sci Transl Med 5:178ra41

3.4.4

Ahmad NN, Pfalzer A, Kaplan LM (2013) Roux-en-Y gastric bypass normalizes the blunted postprandial bile acid excursion associated with obesity. Int J Obes 37:1553–1559

Kohli R, Bradley D, Setchell KD et al (2013) Weight loss induced by Rouy-en-Y gastric bypass but not laparoscopic adjustable gastric banding increases circulating bile acid. J Clin Endocrinol Metab 98:E708–E712

Nguyen A, Bouscarel B (2008) Bile acids and signal transduction: role in glucose homeostasis. Cell Signal 20:2180–2197

Patti ME, Houten SM, Bianco AC et al (2009) Serum bile acids are higher in humans with prior gastric bypass: potential contribution to improved glucose and lipid metabolism. Obesity 17:1671–1677

Metabolic Surgery

J. Ordemann and U. Elbelt

Contents

© Springer-Verlag GmbH Germany, part of Springer Nature 2022
J. Ordemann, U. Elbelt (eds.), *Obesity and Metabolic Surgery*,
https://doi.org/10.1007/978-3-662-63227-7_4

4

The efficacy of bariatric or metabolic surgery in the treatment of type 2 diabetes has been demonstrated beyond doubt in several studies. Thus, metabolic surgery has proven to be an important pillar in the therapy of type 2 diabetes.

More than half a century ago, Friedmann et al. (1955) in New York recognized that gastric surgery had a positive effect on the glucose control of diabetic patients. The term "metabolic surgery" was first introduced by Buchwald and Varco (1978) in the 1970s. More than 20 years ago, Pories et al. (1995) described the pronounced effects of metabolic surgery in an observational study titled, "Who would have thought it?"

In 2014, the British National Institute for Health and Care Excellence (NICE, ► www.nice.org.uk) recommended, taking into account quality of life, lifespan and avoidance of long-term complications of type 2 diabetes, that metabolic surgery should be more accessible to obese patients with diabetes. For health and economic considerations, this surgical therapy option should be made available to more patients. This assessment leads to the assumption that metabolic surgery will also be given a higher priority in the treatment of type 2 diabetes in Germany in the future.

The mechanisms of action of surgical procedures have an indirect and direct influence on the metabolism, which is described in detail in ► Sect. 3.5.

4.1 Prospective Studies

In 2008, a prospective randomized study by Dixon et al. (2008), which demonstrated a significantly stronger influence of the gastric band on glucose control in patients with type 2 diabetes compared to the conservative treatment strategy, was published for the first time. In 2012, two additional prospective randomized studies were published simultaneously in the New England Journal of Medicine. Schauer et al. (2012) treated 150 patients with inadequately controlled type 2 diabetes (HbA$_{1c}$ average 9.2 ± 1.5%). One third of the patients received intensive drug therapy, another third received laparoscopic gastric

bypass, and the last third received laparoscopic sleeve gastrectomy. One year after surgery, 42% of the patients who received gastric bypass showed a remission of type 2 diabetes (defined as HbA$_{1c}$ ≤ 6% without taking diabetic medication), 27% who received sleeve gastrectomy achieved a remission of diabetes and no patients in the conservatively treated group achieved a remission of diabetes. In the course of 3 years the results were impressively confirmed (Schauer et al. 2014). In the bariatric group, the HbA$_{1c}$ value dropped from an average of 9.3–6.7% (gastric bypass) and from 9.5–7.0% (sleeve gastrectomy). In the conservative group, the reduction of the HbA$_{1c}$ value (from 9.0% to 8.4%) was significantly less. The rate of persistent diabetes remission was 35% for patients after gastric bypass and 20% for patients after sleeve gastrectomy. Weight loss was 4.2% in the group that received drug therapy, 24.5% after bypass surgery and 21.1% after sleeve gastrectomy. In terms of fat metabolism, there was a significant increase in HDL cholesterol after 3 years of treatment, 34.7% after gastric bypass and 35.0% after sleeve gastrectomy, compared to 4.6% in the group that received drug therapy. The decrease in triglyceride levels were significantly more pronounced in the gastric bypass group (45.9%) and the sleeve gastrectomy group (31.5%) compared to the group that received drug therapy (21.5%).

Blood pressure was virtually unchanged in all groups, although the reduction of the need for antihypertensive medication after surgery should be noted. An improved quality of life was achieved in the patients who received surgery in terms of health and fitness.

In a long-term study by Brethauer et al. (2013), different bariatric interventions and their effectiveness on the diabetic metabolic situation were compared over a 6-year period. In this study 217 patients were examined: 162 patients received a gastric bypass, 23 a sleeve gastrectomy and 32 a gastric band. The best results in terms of diabetes remission were achieved by patients who received gastric bypass.

The pronounced metabolic effect of biliopancreatic diversion was demonstrated by Mingrone et al. (2012) in a prospective randomized study. In this study, 60 higher-grade obese patients with type 2 diabetes were examined. 20 patients received biliopancreatic diversion, another 20 received gastric bypass, and 20 patients underwent optimized drug therapy. Two years after surgery, the authors documented a remission of type 2 diabetes in 95% of patients after biliopancreatic diversion and in 75% after bypass surgery. Patients who received conservative therapy did not achieve remission.

The Swedish Obese Subjects (SOS) study initiated almost 30 years ago by Sjöström et al. (2014) shows comparable results with a diabetes reemission rate of 72% two years after surgery compared to 16% in the control group. After 15 years, the number of patients in remission was reduced to 30%, but it was still much higher than in the conservative therapy group with 6%, although at that time restrictive procedures such as the gastric band were largely in use.

4.2 Meta-Analyses

Buchwald et al. (2009) showed in a meta-analysis the significant influence of metabolic surgery on type 2 diabetes. 82% of the patients showed an improvement in glucose control within the first 2 years after surgery, and 62% were in remission for more than 2 years. The most pronounced influence on diabetes remission within 2 years was biliopancreatic diversion (94%), followed by gastric bypass (82%), gastroplasty (81%) and finally gastric banding (55%). This meta-analysis included publications from 1990 to 2006, which involved a total of 135,246 patients.

A more recent meta-analysis by Chang et al. (2014) included 37 randomized studies and 127 observational studies from 2003 to 2012. Gastric bypass and sleeve gastrectomy proved to be similarly effective in the treatment of type 2 diabetes. The meta-analysis by Zhang et al. (2014), also published in 2014, compares the 2-year results after gastric bypass and sleeve gastrectomy on the basis of 16 studies with 9756 patients. Gastric bypass led to more pronounced weight reduction, but there was no significant difference between gastric bypass and sleeve gastrectomy in terms of metabolic control of type 2 diabetes.

Another meta-analysis by Parikh et al. (2013) compared the different surgical procedures in patients with a BMI of <35 kg/m². This analysis confirmed the results of the meta-analyses which was carried out up to then for type 2 diabetes with low obesity: In the surgical group an improvement in glucose control was documented in 95% of the patients, 55% of the patients even achieved a remission of their type 2 diabetes. The patient group after biliopancreatic diversion showed the most favourable results.

Overall, the available data demonstrates that the more invasive the procedure, the more impressive the success in terms of weight reduction and glucose control. The gastric band shows the least effect on type 2 diabetes, and the restriction alone does not allow a direct metabolic effect. This is achieved indirectly over time by weight reduction. The most pronounced effect on blood glucose control can be observed after biliopancreatic diversion (with or without duodenal switch). The remission rates are very high and weight reduction is also the most pronounced. However, the rates on complication are also the highest. In comparison, gastric bypass and sleeve gastrectomy show similarly good therapeutic effects with a low rate of complication. Both methods seem to offer the most impressive results in the risk-benefit assessment, with the gastric bypass tending to have a more pronounced effect on blood sugar regulation than the sleeve gastrectomy.

4.3 Postoperative Incidence of Diabetes, Micro- and Macrovascular Complications, Life Expectancy

In the SOS study (2012), new cases of diabetes after bariatric surgery occurred significantly less frequently than in the patients who did not receive surgery, with rates of 1% vs. 8% after 2 years and 7% vs. 24% after 10 years. Moreover, in the 15-year evaluation (Sjöström et al. 2014), the cumulative incidence of micro-

4

vascular complications was reduced by half (42 events per 1000 years in the control group vs. 21 events per 1000 years in the patients who received surgery) and that of macrovascular complications was reduced by about one quarter (44 events per 1000 years in the control group vs. 32 events per 1000 years in the patients who received surgery). Thus, the development of diabetes-related microvascular damage to kidneys, eyes and nerves can be slowed down and even prevented by metabolic surgery.

> **Practical Tip**
>
> Regular ophthalmological check-ups must be ensured even after achieving a diabetes remission. A diabetic retinopathy or its worsening can also occur postoperatively.

Long-term studies, such as the SOS study, show significant survival benefits from obesity surgery. An analysis of US-American databases (Schauer et al. 2015) involving approximately 200,000 patients shows this for the first time specifically under the aspect of "metabolic surgery and life expectancy": Below a BMI of 62 kg/m^2, all type 2 diabetics seem to benefit dramatically from a metabolic intervention, regardless of gender and weight. The remaining life expectancy of a 45-year-old obese type 2 diabetic is extended from 31.7 to 38.4 years.

As far as quality of life is concerned, the results have not yet been so convincingly confirmed by studies. In particular, the frequency of occurrence of postbariatric hyperinsulinemic hypoglycaemic syndrome (▶ Sect. 14.8.1) needs to be investigated more closely.

❶ It is important to note that the evaluation of the effect of bariatric surgery on metabolic control in type 1 diabetes using the parameters of weight progression and HbA_{1c} reduction which are usually recorded in studies is insufficient.

In particular, surgical procedures with abolition of the delayed passage of food into the small intestine through the pylorus consid-

erably complicate a safe metabolic situation and are accompanied by pronounced, rapidly changing blood sugar fluctuations which are difficult to counteract therapeutically.

> **Conclusion**
>
> The available clinical studies underline the superiority of surgical therapy of type 2 diabetes compared to conservative therapy.
>
> The more intensive the surgical intervention is, the more successful is not only the weight reduction, but also the remission rate of the diabetes disease. The available data show that remission rates are lower for the gastric band than for other metabolic interventions, that gastric bypass tends to get better results than sleeve gastrectomy, and that biliopancreatic diversion has the highest rates of remission.
>
> In Germany sleeve gastrectomy, gastric bypass, gastric banding and biliopancreatic diversion are considered standard procedures, with sleeve gastrectomy and gastric bypass accounting for about 95% of the procedures. According to the risk-benefit assessment, both procedures lead to favourable weight reduction and metabolic improvement.

References

Brethauer SA, Aminian A, Romero-Talamas H et al (2013) Can diabetes be surgically cured? Long-term metabolic effects of bariatric surgery in obese patients with type 2 diabetes mellitus. Ann Surg 258:628–636

Buchwald H, Avidor Y, Braunwald E et al (2009) Weight and type 2 diabetes after bariatric surgery: systematic review and meta-analysis. Am J Med 122:248–256

Buchwald H, Varco RL (1978) Metabolic surgery. Grune and Stratton, New York

Chang SH, Stoll CR, Song J et al (2014) The effectiveness and risks of bariatric surgery: an updated systematic review and meta-analysis, 2003–2012. JAMA Surg 149:275–287

Dixon JB, O'Brien PE, Playfair J et al (2008) Adjustable gastric banding and conventional therapy for type 2 diabetes: a randomized controlled trial. JAMA 299:316–323

Friedman MN, Sancetta AJ, Magovern GJ (1955) The amelioration of diabetes mellitus following subtotal gastrectomy. Surg Gynecol Obstet 100:201–204

Mingrone G, Panunzi S, De Gaetano A et al (2012) Bariatric surgery versus conventional medical therapy for type 2 diabetes. N Engl J Med 366:1577–1585

Parikh M, Issa R, Vieira D et al (2013) Role of bariatric surgery as treatment for type 2 diabetes in patients who do not meet current NIH criteria: a systematic review and meta-analysis. J Am Coll Surg 217: 527–532

Pories WJ, Swanson MS, MacDonald KG et al (1995) Who would have thought it? An operation proves to be the most effective therapy for adult-onset diabetes mellitus. Ann Surg 222:339–350

Schauer DP, Arterburn DE, Livingston EH et al (2015) Impact of bariatric surgery on life expectancy in severely obese patients with diabetes: a decision analysis. Ann Surg 261:914–919

Schauer PR, Bhatt DL, Kirwan JP et al (2014) Bariatric surgery versus intensive medical therapy for diabetes – 3 year outcomes. N Engl J Med 370:2002–2013

Schauer PR, Kashyap SR, Wolski K et al (2012) Bariatric surgery versus intensive medical therapy in obese patients with diabetes. N Engl J Med 366: 1567–1576

Sjöström L, Peltonen M, Jacobson P et al (2014) Association of bariatric surgery with long-term remission of type 2 diabetes and with microvascular and macrovascular complications. JAMA 311: 2297–2304

Zhang C, Yuan Y, Qiu C, Zhang W (2014) A meta-analysis of 2 year effect after surgery: laparoscopic Roux-en-Y gastric bypass versus laparoscopic sleeve gastrectomy for morbid obesity and diabetes mellitus. Obes Surg 24:1528–1535

Further Readings

Blüher M (2014) Insulin oder Chirurgie? Die Sicht des Diabetologen. Chirurg 85:957–962

Carlsson LM, Peltonen M, Ahlin S et al (2012) Bariatric surgery and prevention of type 2 diabetes in Swedish obese subjects. N Engl J Med 367:695–704

Hedberg J, Sundström J, Sundbom M (2014) Duodenal switch versus Roux-en-Y gastric bypass for morbid obesity: systematic review and meta-analysis of weight results, diabetes resolution and early complications in single-centre comparisons. Obes Rev 15:555–563

Hüttl TP, Kramer KM, Wood H (2010) Bariatrische Chirurgie—Adipositaschirurgische Verfahren und ihre Besonderheiten. Diabetologe 8:637–646

Hüttl TP, Stauch P, Wood H, Fruhmann J (2015) Bariatrische Chirurgie. Aktuelle Ernährungsmed 40:256–274

Miras AD, le Roux CW (2014) Metabolic surgery: shifting the focus from glycaemia and weight to end-organ health. Lancet Diabetes Endocrinol 2:141–151

Peterli R, Steinert RE, Woelnerhanssen B et al (2012) Metabolic and hormonal changes after laparoscopic Roux-en-Y gastric bypass and sleeve gastrectomy: a randomized, prospective trial. Obes Surg 22:740 748

Runkel N, Colombo-Benkmann M, Hüttl TP et al (2011) Bariatric surgery. Dtsch Arztebl Int 108:341–346

Sjöström L, Narbro K, Sjöström CD et al (2007) Effect of bariatric surgery on mortality in Swedish obese subjects. N Engl J Med 357:741–752

Preoperative Evaluation of the Patient

J. Ordemann, U. Elbelt, and T. Hofmann

Contents

© Springer-Verlag GmbH Germany, part of Springer Nature 2022
J. Ordemann, U. Elbelt (eds.), *Obesity and Metabolic Surgery*,
https://doi.org/10.1007/978-3-662-63227-7_5

5.1 Surgical Evaluation

J. Ordemann

The foundations of many interdisciplinary obesity centres were predominantly initiated by bariatric surgeons. The surgical presentation is often the first contact of the patient at the interdisciplinary obesity centre. Surgical indication, contraindications, assessment of the surgical risk and education are elementary components of the surgical evaluation. In addition, the coordination of the necessary interdisciplinary evaluation, patient support and assistance in applying for cost coverage are also important. In the future, these organisational tasks will increasingly be transferred to internists.

The following questions have to be clarified by surgical evaluation:
- Is there a pathological overweight?
- Which concomitant diseases are present?
- Which therapeutic goals are to be achieved?
- Have conservative therapies already been carried out?
- How high is the risk of an operation?
- Which procedure is applicable?
- Is regular aftercare possible?

The surgical evaluation includes a detailed anamnesis and the assessment of potential surgical contraindications. Since obesity can affect practically every organ system, a physical examination must be performed in addition to the medical history. Pre-surgery, gastroesophageal reflux, tumour diseases, allergies and the patient's ability to cooperate have to also be evaluated. If significant risk factors and concomitant diseases are present, early presentation to the anaesthesiologist is recommended. The surgical presentation also includes information of the patient about the possible surgical procedures.

The surgeon should initially decide against surgery if the following contraindications are present—they are listed in the S3 guidelines:
- insufficient conservative therapy attempts,
- active malignant tumours,
- chronic substance abuse,
- florid psychiatric diseases,
- advanced cirrhosis of the liver,
- insufficient cooperation of the patient,
- pregnancy.

In the context of evaluation, it should be noted that the classification of obesity by BMI is inadequate. BMI is not the only decisive factor for the therapy decision. In particular, comorbidities such as diabetes mellitus type 2, arterial hypertension, cardiovascular disease, orthopaedic diseases, depression and behaviour (especially eating behaviour) have to be considered.

For assessment purposes, the classification according to Sharma and Kushner (2009), the so-called Edmonton Obesity Staging System (EOSS), has been established (◘ Fig. 5.1). This classification was developed in order to document the disease burden of obesity in addition to the BMI. The EOSS allows an individual-

◘ **Fig. 5.1** The Edmonton Obesity Staging System according to Sharma and Kushner. (From Sharma and Kushner 2009, with kind permission)

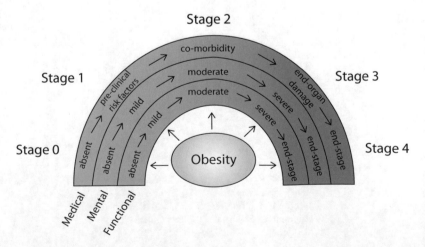

ized assessment taking into account relevant concomitant diseases and should therefore be consistently applied in surgical evaluations.

It consists of five stages:

- **Stage 0**

There are no risk factors associated with obesity, no physical symptoms, no psychopathology, no functional limitations or impairment of well-being.

- **Stage 1**

There are: one or more obesity-associated risk factors of subclinical severity (e.g. impaired fasting glucose, labile arterial hypertension), mild physical symptoms such as shortness of breath during moderate physical activity, mild psychopathological symptoms or a slight impairment of well-being.

- **Stage 2**

The patient has one or more manifest obesity-related diseases requiring medical treatment (arterial hypertension, diabetes mellitus type 2, polycystic ovary syndrome, anxiety disorder).

- **Stage 3**

The patient has clinically significant end organ damage such as myocardial infarction, cardiac insufficiency, complications of type 2 diabetes mellitus as well as significant functional limitations and limitations in well-being.

- **Stage 4**

The patient suffers from advanced end organ damage due to obesity-related comorbidities, severe psychopathologies and serious impairment of well-being.

> ❶ However, the EOSS does not allow any conclusions to be drawn about the specific operational risk and does not replace the anaesthesiological risk assessment.

The surgical evaluation is completed by combining the findings and taking into account the endocrinological and psychosomatic evaluation and therapeutic recommendations. This very time-consuming, mostly outpatient procedure requires several diagnostic visits.

5.2　Internal Evaluation

U. Elbelt

The task of preoperative internal examination is to identify syndromic forms of obesity or endocrinological diseases leading to obesity. Furthermore, comorbidities associated with obesity have to be diagnosed and appropriate drug therapy has to be initiated. Furthermore, a preoperative lack of macro- or micronutrients has to be detected and compensated.

The hereditary obesity is rare. The development of obesity in early childhood in conjunction with accompanying endocrine disorders is indicative (❏ Fig. 5.2). The causes are homozygous mutations in the leptin or leptin receptor gene or genetic defects in the downstream leptin-melanocortin signalling path-

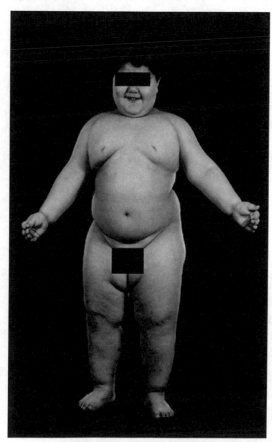

3yr old weighing 42 kg

❏ **Fig. 5.2**　Child with leptin deficiency

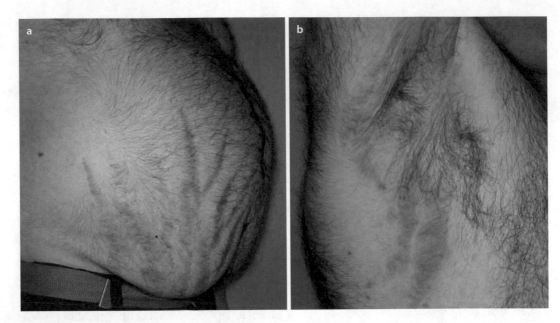

Fig. 5.3 **a, b** Skin manifestations of hypercortisolism

way (mutations in the proopiomelanocortin [POMC], prohormone convertase 1 [PC1], melanocortin-4-receptor [MC4R] gene). Other hereditary syndromes associated with obesity are mostly characterised by indicative features of the face and hands, hypogonadism and mental retardation (e.g., Prader-Willi syndrome, Laurence-Moon-Biedl). The diagnosis is nearly always made in childhood.

The internal preoperative assessment of adult patients prior to bariatric surgery should include thyroid function testing (determination of basal TSH), whereby the influence of mildly acquired hypothyroidism on the development of obesity is often overestimated.

> **Practical Tip**
>
> The preoperative exclusion of Cushing's syndrome, which leads to weight gain, impaired glucose tolerance and arterial hypertension, is of high clinical relevance.

During the clinical examination, attention should be paid to signs and symptoms of Cushing's syndrome, in particular truncal obesity in the presence of thin limbs, easy bruising and reddish-purple stretch marks (Striae rubrae distensae) more than 1 cm

wide (■ Fig. 5.3). It is also helpful to ask the patients to stand up from a squatting position. While this is usually possible at least once for obese patients, patients with Cushing's syndrome usually do not succeed. They often have to help themselves with their arms because of the proximal muscle weakness. The prevalence is about 1% in patients who intend to undergo bariatric surgery. Differential diagnosis is particularly difficult in patients with mild Cushing's syndrome. Routine screening (in contrast to the previous guidelines) therefore appears to be absolutely necessary in view of the relevance for further therapeutic decisions. The benefit for the affected patients is high, since treatment can reduce the increased morbidity and mortality caused by hypercortisolism, prevent perioperative complications (especially thromboembolism) and detect malignant diseases that may lead to hypercortisolism at an early stage.

For diagnosis, a dexamethasone suppression test should be performed primarily. The patient takes 1 mg of dexamethasone around 11 pm. The next morning at about 8 am the concentration of cortisol in serum is measured. Alternatively, a 24-h urine sampling can be carried out twice to quantify free cortisol excretion or midnight salivary cortisol can be determined twice.

In the case of rapid weight gain in connection with a change in character, tumours and inflammations in the area of the hypothalamus should be considered (e.g. craniopharyngioma).

In addition to the determination of the BMI, the waist-hip ratio, which is used to estimate visceral obesity, should be determined to identify high-risk patients with regard to the occurrence of cardiovascular disease. Furthermore, a thorough anamnesis with regard to additional cardiovascular risk factors is necessary and corresponding diagnostic investigations should be initiated. In addition, clinical signs of insulin resistance should be looked for, such as a dorsocervical fat pad and skin changes (hyperpigmentation and hyperkeratosis) of the neck and axillary region known as acanthosis nigricans benigna (■ Fig. 5.4).

Furthermore, HbA_{1c} and blood glucose are measured. In case of diagnostic uncertainty, an oral glucose tolerance test should be performed with a low threshold. The blood pressure should be measured repeatedly and, if necessary, an outpatient 24-h blood pressure measurement should be performed. If cardiovascular risk factors are present, their consistent treatment is necessary. Especially for antidiabetic therapy, substances that do not promote further weight gain should be preferred (metformin, incretin-based therapies). In addition, pre-existing cardiovascular complications (cardiac insufficiency, angina pectoris, coronary heart disease, myocardial infarction, peripheral arterial occlusive disease, cerebrovascular insufficiency) have to be carefully inquired. Screening for the presence of obesity and sleep-related breathing disorders is recommended. In the presence of a sleep apnea syndrome requiring treatment or an obesity hypoventilation syndrome, the initiation of preoperative nocturnal continuous positive airway pressure ventilation is recommended.

> **Practical Tip**
>
> In the context of a careful drug anamnesis, the possibility of changing drug therapies promoting weight gain, such as most antidepressants, antipsychotics, anticonvulsants, glucocorticoids and beta blockers, should be assessed.

Medical history and physical examination should focus on the identification of nutritional deficiencies, especially with regard to micronutrients. Recommended preoperative laboratory diagnostics are shown in ■ Table 5.1. Diag-

■ **Table 5.1** Recommended preoperative testing	
Lipid status	Total, LDL, HDL cholesterol, triglycerides
Glucose control	Fasting blood glucose, HbA_{1c} (possibly OGTT)
Endocrinology	TSH (possibly fT3, fT4), cortisol in the dexamethasone suppression test, (alternatively: cortisol in the 24-h urine sampling or midnight saliva cortisol)
Screening for nutrient deficiencies	BB, vitamin D3 (possibly PTH, vitamin B12, folic acid and iron status)
Routine	Liver enzymes, cholestatic parameters, renal retention parameters, PTT/INR, electrolytes, calcium
Instrumental diagnostics	ECG, sonography of the abdomen, gastroscopy (possibly X-ray thorax, DXA)

DXA Dual-X-Ray absorptiometry

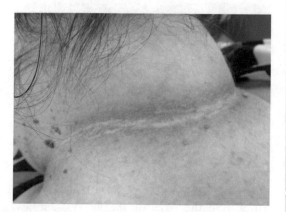

■ **Fig. 5.4** Cervical acanthosis nigricans benigna

nosed nutrient deficiencies must be compensated for prior to the operation (▶ Sect. 14.5).

As a rule, prior to intended bariatric surgery, an electrocardiogram should be recorded and patients should undergo esophagogastroduodenoscopy to exclude ulcers and malignancies as well as sonography of the abdomen to rule out the presence of gallstones and to estimate the size of the liver. In women, bone mineral density of the lumbar spine (L1–L4) and/or proximal femur using Dual-X-Ray Absorptiometry (DXA) should be assessed with a low threshold.

In addition to the internal evaluation, a detailed dietary history should be taken by a nutritionist, if possible. The following points should be recorded in order to enable an assessment of eating behaviour (adapted from Freedhoff and Sharma 2012):

- Meal frequency,
- Composition of the meal,
- Quantity of food consumed during and between meals, energy intake,
- Asking about hunger and satiety,
- Survey the eating habits (e.g. alone, in company, at home, out of town),
- Emotional experiences related to food,
- Prior experience with diets.

5.3 Psychosomatic Evaluation

T. Hofmann

The S3 guideline on obesity surgery recommends preoperative psychosomatic, psychological or psychiatric evaluation. This recommendation is based on the knowledge of a significant psychosocial comorbidity in this group, in which up to 70% of all patients have been affected by a manifest mental disorder in their lifetime.

The psychosomatic evaluation is primarily carried out in the form of direct personal interviews; psychometric questionnaires are also used. In particular, the patient's medical history and current status with regard to mental illness and other psychosocial limitations should be questioned (◻ Table 5.2). Special attention should be paid in the anamnesis to suicide attempts or suicidal thoughts, as well as to the use or abuse of substances and to behavioural addictions in the previous history. In addition, information on eating behaviour is important in order to identify eating disorders. The knowledge of previous weight history and its relation to life events may be indicative for the latter. The chances of success of conservative weight reduction can be estimated by assessment of previous weight loss or dietary experience. In addition, the knowledge of the patient's body image is relevant in order to anticipate possible difficulties in dealing with the post-operatively altered body.

Furthermore, the expectations of the operation should be discussed in detail with the patients. It is not uncommon for surgical procedures to be associated with excessively high expectations regarding weight loss and the aesthetics of physical changes; the surgical treatment is sometimes seen as a kind of quick and comprehensive solution to all problems that are one-sidedly attributed to high body weight. In addition, cognitive functions and personality structure should be assessed, as these can also have an impact on the post-operative outcome.

Further important topics are the fundamental willingness to change previous lifestyle and nutritional habits, as well as adherence to the lifelong treatment necessary even after bariatric surgery in the form of regular medical follow-ups including possible substitution of vitamins and micronutrients.

> **Practical Tip**
>
> Indications of the postoperative expected therapeutic adherence in postoperative care can be drawn from the handling of previous medical recommendations and the adherence to long-term medication.

It may be advantageous to carry out the psychosomatic evaluation after the surgical and internal presentation, if the patients are already informed about the differential indication and the risks of the various surgical

◻ Table 5.2 Elements of a psychosomatic evaluation prior to a planned bariatric operation

Psychic status	Psychological findings incl. body image perception Biographical anamnesis History of mental illnesses and their treatment including psychopharmacological medication Special attention to suicidal crises and addictions
Social situation	Evaluation of current psychosocial stress and social support
Somatic status	General somatic medical history Presence of pre-existing obesity-related diseases Current medication
Family anamnesis	Familial occurrence of obesity or other weight disorders Family history of eating disorders, depression, anxiety disorders
Individual weight course	Anamnesis of the course of weight within the previous life span (incl. possible context to life events) History of previous self-directed and professionally supported weight reduction attempts
Eating and nutritional behaviour	Eating habits including food and drink selection, meal structure and rhythm (e.g. skipping meals) Occurrence and frequency of hunger pangs Occurrence of emotionally triggered eating, grazing, sweet eating, night eating Counter-regulatory behaviour (food restriction, vomiting, laxatives, appetite suppressants, sport as counter-regulation)
Motivation and adherence to therapy	Subjective motivation for a surgical treatment Expectations regarding the outcome of the operation (extent of weight loss and its influence on individual life: Is the operation considered a simple solution to pre-existing problems)? Motivation for multimodal treatment of obesity (preparative/accompanying) Willingness for postoperative psychosomatic support Dealing with previous medical treatments
Knowledge of the therapeutic procedure	Knowledge about the planned operation Knowledge of operational risks Knowledge of the need for postoperative dietary changes Knowledge about the necessity of (lifelong) post-operative aftercare, including vitamin and micronutrient supplementation that may become necessary Knowledge of the psychological course to be expected postoperatively and the risks regarding suicidal tendencies and substance abuse

Adapted from Müller et al. (2012)

procedures and if endocrinological causes of obesity have been excluded. At this point, the patients' understanding of the often complex procedure can be better assessed. In addition, concepts that integrate surgical, endocrinological and psychosomatic evaluation and coordinate them in a timely manner appear advantageous.

On the basis of current empirical data, mental disorders or certain personality traits per se do not constitute a contraindication for bariatric surgery. Only unstable psychopathological states such as psychoses, suicidal tendencies, active substance addictions or an untreated bulimia nervosa are regarded as contraindications. In addition, if major difficulties are to be expected, the pros and cons of a surgical procedure should be weighed up with regard to the reliable adherence to necessary surgical aftercare and a required vitamin supplementation. Also, the severity and especially the handling of patients with mental disorders such as depression or anxiety disorders seem to be of importance. Depression or anxiety disorders already present preoperatively may indicate a lower postoperative weight loss, which is, however, generally still clinically significant. Therefore, the presence of depression or anxiety disorders is an indication for their professional treatment, but not a contraindication for bariatric surgery.

Patients who suffer preoperatively from hunger pangs, for example in the context of a binge-eating disorder (see ▶ Sect. 1.6), cannot be expected to experience less weight loss after bariatric surgery per se. However, postoperative hunger pangs in the sense of loss-of-control-eating (defined as the experience of a loss of control over food regardless of the amount of food eaten) are more frequent, which in turn may be associated with a lower postoperative weight loss.

In the presence of a mental disorder, adequate psychotherapeutic and drug treatment should therefore be initiated before the operation in order to achieve the most favourable starting position possible at the time of the surgical procedure. In the case of more severe or unstable mental disorders, re-evaluation with regard to bariatric surgery should take place after stabilization.

Another important function of preoperative evaluation is to inform patients about the importance of adequate psychosomatic aftercare. Depending on the degree of risk, a regular presentation should be discussed due to the unfavourable influence of, for example, depressive disorders or newly occurring hunger pangs on the surgical outcome. This can take place, for example, contemporaneous to surgical and internal aftercare appointments; alternatively, it can also be arranged at the discretion of the patient only when psychological problems arise.

The psychosomatic evaluation therefore has less of a "gatekeeper" function, but should rather serve, in addition to the identification of mental disorders requiring treatment, to optimise the postoperative outcome in terms of weight loss and quality of life, and also to prepare patients for the psychosocial changes and demands after bariatric surgery. Under no circumstances should the psychosomatic evaluation result in a disadvantage for patients with mental disorders or obese patients whose treatment adherence is limited. These patients should not be deprived of an indicated surgical procedure. For a psychosomatic optimisation of the postoperative course, however, many centres currently still lack a differentiated offer, ranging from simple and one-off psychosomatic evaluation to multimodal therapy programmes and full psychotherapeutic treatment.

5.4　Choice of Procedure

J. Ordemann

A surgical gold standard in bariatric surgery does not exist. Numerous factors such as weight, age, concomitant diseases, psychosocial stress, social environment and preference influence the decision-making process. The choice of the surgical procedure should be discussed in detail with the patient and should be a shared and individual decision. The advantages and disadvantages of the different procedures have to be discussed with the patient in detail.

For the choice of procedure, the following questions have to be answered:
1. What is the initial weight?
2. What expectations does the patient have in regard to the operation?
3. What is the patient's previous eating behaviour?
4. What is the risk profile of the patient?
5. How pronounced is the weight loss to be expected from the bariatric intervention?
6. Which procedure has the strongest influence on the patient's comorbidities, in particular on diabetes mellitus type 2?
7. What is the patient's adherence to therapy?

The patient's cooperation can be assessed on the basis of previous diets and participation in exercise programmes. In addition, age, occupation, medication (anticoagulants, immunosuppressants) and social environment play a role in the decision for or against a specific bariatric procedure.

The patient's understanding of the different mechanisms of action of the different surgical procedures should also be taken into account. The patient should know that restriction and malabsorption after bariatric surgery allow weight loss, but that specific hormonal and neuronal postoperative changes also play a role.

The choice of procedure for the surgical intervention can be individualised by interdisciplinary assessment (surgeon, internist, psychosomatics specialist, nutritional therapist) within the framework of an "obesity board". The wish of the often well-informed patients regarding the surgical procedure has to be considered for the decision-making process. On principal, obesity surgery operations should be performed laparoscopically.

The following recommendations are usually made with regard to eating behaviour:

— Restrictive procedures are recommended for patients with "hyperphagic eating behaviour", who eat larger meals and hardly feel any sense of satiety. Sleeve gastrectomy seems to be particularly suitable here.
— Patients who frequently and regularly take snacks ("snackers") are recommended to undergo a gastric bypass.
— Patients who are more likely to consume sweets or sugary drinks ("sweet eaters") are also recommended to undergo a gastric bypass or a biliopancreatic diversion.

In addition to the consideration of eating habits, comorbidities, especially type 2 diabetes mellitus, have to be taken into account. Apart from weight reduction, the improvement of concomitant and secondary diseases is of major relevance for the choice of the surgical procedure.

It has been shown that with increasing complexity of the surgical procedure (biliopancreatic diversion > gastric bypass > sleeve gastrectomy > gastric banding), blood glucose control and the remission rate of diabetes mellitus type 2 improve. Gastric banding, if at all, should play a minor role in the treatment of obesity and diabetes mellitus type 2 and should only be recommended in individual cases. The mere restriction due to the gastric band does not allow a convincing metabolic effect. Compared to gastric banding, gastric bypass and sleeve gastrectomy lead to more effective blood sugar control and higher diabetes mellitus type 2 remission rates. Gastric bypass tends to be superior to

sleeve gastrectomy in this respect (▶ Chap. 4). Biliopancreatic diversion has the greatest effect on blood glucose control and diabetes remission. However, the higher peri- and postoperative complication rate must be taken into account, because parallel to the metabolic effectiveness, the complication rate increases with the increasing complexity of the bariatric intervention.

Although sleeve gastrectomy has a lower complication rate compared to gastric bypass, the possible development of gastroesophageal reflux disease has to be taken into account. Therefore, a pre-existing reflux disease of the patient as well as a hiatus hernia should be assessed in the preoperative evaluation. A symptomatic hiatus hernia represents a relative contraindication for sleeve gastrectomy.

In order to reduce the perioperative risk in patients with extreme obesity or considerable comorbidity, a two-stage concept (step-by-step concept) can be considered (▶ Chap. 16). One example would be the placement of a gastric balloon. The short-term weight reduction achieved by this can lead to a reduction in comorbidities and thus to a reduction in perioperative mortality. In addition, the intraoperative conditions can improve significantly, for example in the form of a smaller liver volume. The sleeve gastrectomy as the first intervention of a biliopancreatic diversion with duodenal switch is also considered a classic two-stage concept.

5.5 Informing the Patient

J. Ordemann

As with any surgical intervention, the principle applies in obesity surgery that a curative surgical intervention legally constitutes bodily injury. Therefore, effective consent is required as a justification.

The obesity surgeon is obliged to provide comprehensive and timely information. Patients who wish to undergo bariatric surgery have to be informed about the scope and importance of the procedure. The aim of the educational discussion is not only to inform about the course of the procedure but also about the possible risks and consequences of the intervention (see below). The information has to be documented in writing. Sketches and individual remarks improve counselling and increase its credibility. The documentation does not replace the educational discussion with the patient. The consent form has to be signed by the patient as well as by the doctor providing the information.

In general, it is recommended that the surgeon performing the surgery also provides information. The decisive factor is that the informing person is sufficiently skilled for discussing all relevant issues with the patient.

Prior to all bariatric interventions it should be pointed out that obesity is a chronic disease and the surgical intervention is to be regarded as an "attempt to cure". The surgical intervention is to be understood as one component of an interdisciplinary overall concept of obesity therapy and requires a comprehensive change of life and lifelong aftercare. Furthermore, the necessity of supplementation with vitamins and micronutrients has to be highlighted. In addition, especially in the case of malabsorptive procedures, attention should be drawn to possible changes in the effectiveness of drugs (e.g., loss of efficacy of oral contraceptives). Moreover, information on potential revision procedures and the potential necessity of follow-up operations (plastic surgery) is part of the patient education and counselling.

> **Practical Tip**
>
> Patient education should comprise the discussion of treatment alternatives (conservative obesity therapy) and this should be documented carefully.

Information must be provided in good time before the procedure so that the patient has sufficient time to reconsider his decision. Since bariatric procedures are elective procedures, it is recommended that the patient is informed to the time when the appointment for the surgical procedure is made. If the time period between providing information and the operation is too long, it is advisable to repeat the patient education shortly before the operation.

In addition to the general risks of an operation, information must be provided about the specific risks of the various bariatric surgical procedures:

▪ **Gastric Banding**

Placement of a foreign body. Risks: Injuries to the stomach or oesophagus, material damage, catheter breakage, port defect, infections, slippage of the gastric band, intolerance, migration of the gastric band, less weight loss compared to other bariatric surgical procedures.

▪ **Sleeve Gastrectomy**

Irreversible intervention. Risks: Suture insufficiency, peritonitis, gastric sleeve dilatation, reflux and heartburn, stenosis. Need for supplementation.

▪ **Gastric Bypass**

Risks: Dumping, dilatation of the gastric pouch, suture insufficiency, peritonitis, internal hernia, stenosis of the anastomoses. Need for supplementation.

▪ **Omega Loop Bypass**

Risks: Suture insufficiency, peritonitis, bile-acid reflux, stenosis. Need for supplementation.

▪ **BPD According to Scopinaro/BPD with DS**

Risks: Suture insufficiency, peritonitis, hernias, stenosis of the anastomoses, fatty stools and gastrointestinal complaints, dilatation of the gastric pouch (BPD with duodenal switch). Need for supplementation.

References

5.1

Sharma AM, Kushner RF (2009) A proposed clinical staging system for obesity. Int J Obes 33:289–295

5.2

Freedhoff Y, Sharma AM, Hellbardt M, Schilling-Maßmann B, Haberl PM (2012) Best weight. Ein Leitfaden für das Adipositas-Management. Pabst Science Publishers, Lengerich

5.3

Müller A, Herpertz S, de Zwaan M (2012) Psychosomatische Aspekte der Adipositaschirurgie. Psychother Psychosom Med Psychol 62:473–479

Further Readings

5.1

Deutsche Adipositas-Gesellschaft, Deutsche Diabetes Gesellschaft, Deutsche Gesellschaft für Ernährung, deutsche Gesellschaft für Ernährungsmedizin (2014a) Interdisziplinäre Leitlinie der Qualität S3 zur, Prävention und Therapie der Adipositas. AWMF-Register Nr. 050/001. Klasse: S3. Version 2.0. http://www.adipositas-gesellschaft.de/fileadmin/PDF/Leitlinien/S3_Adipositas_Praevention_Therapie_2014.pdf. (25. April 2016)

Deutsche Gesellschaft für Allgemein- und Viszeralchirurgie, Chirurgische Arbeitsgemeinschaft für Adipositastherapie (CAADIP), Deutsche Adipositas-Gesellschft (DAG), Deutsche Gesellschaft für Psychosomatische Medizin und Psychotherapie, Deutsche Gesellschaft für Ernährungsmedizin (2010a) S3-Leitlinie: Chirurgie der Adipositas. http://www.adipositas-gesellschaft.de/fileadmin/PDF/Leitlinien/ADIP-6-2010.pdf. (25. April 2016)

Hüttl TP, Stauch P, Wood H, Fruhmann J (2015) Bariatrische Chirurgie. Aktuelle Ernährungsmed 40:256–274

5.2

Deutsche Adipositas-Gesellschaft, Deutsche Diabetes Gesellschaft, Deutsche Gesellschaft für Ernährung, deutsche Gesellschaft für Ernährungsmedizin (2014b) ► literature 5.1

Deutsche Gesellschaft für Allgemein- und Viszeralchirurgie, Chirurgische Arbeitsgemeinschaft für Adipositastherapie (CAADIP), Deutsche Adipositas-Gesellschaft (DAG), Deutsche Gesellschaft für Psychosomatische Medizin und Psychotherapie, Deutsche Gesellschaft für Ernährungsmedizin (2010b) ► literature 5.1

Farooqi S, O'Rahilly S (2014) 20 Years of Leptin: human disorders of leptin action. J Endocrinology 223: T63–T70

Flier JS, Maratos-Flier E Elbelt U, Scholze JE (2012) Adipositas. In: Longo DL, Fauci AS, Kaspar DL, et al. (Hrsg) Harrisons Innere Medizin, 18. Aufl. ABW Wissenschaftsverlag, Berlin, S 665–672

Fierabracci P, Pinchera A, Martinelli S et al (2011) Prevalence of endocrine diseases in morbidly obese patients scheduled for bariatric surgery: beyond diabetes. Obes Surg 21:54–60

Fried M, Yumuk V, Oppert J-M et al (2013) Interdisciplinary European guidelines on metabolic and baritric surgery. Obes Facts 6:449–468

Kushner RF Elbelt U, Scholze JE (2012) Diagnostik und Management der Adipositas. In: Longo DL, Fauci AS, Kaspar DL, et al. (Hrsg) Harrisons Innere Medizin, 18. Aufl. ABW Wissenschaftsverlag, Berlin, S 673–681

Mechanik JI, Youdim A, Jones DB et al (2013) Clinical practice guidelines for the perioperative nutritional, metabolic, and nonsurgical support of the bariatric surgery patient-2013 Update: cosponsored by American Association of Clinical Endocrinologists, The Obesity Society, and American Society for Metabolic & Bariatric Surgery. Obesity 21:S1–S27

Plewig G, Landthaler M, Burgdorf WHC, Hertl M, Ruzicka T (Hrsg) (2012) Braun-Falco's Dermatologie, Venerologie und Allergologie, 6. Aufl. Springer, Heidelberg

Singh A, Tipton K (2013) Preoperative evaluation of the obese patient. Bariat Surg Pract Pat Care 8:127–133

Wiegand S, Krude H (2015) Monogene und syndromale Krankheitsbilder bei morbider Adipositas. Internist 56:111–120

5.3

Deutsche Gesellschaft für Allgemein- und Viszeralchirurgie, Chirurgische Arbeitsgemeinschaft für Adipositastherapic (CAADIP), Deutsche Adipositas-Gesellschaft (DAG), Deutsche Gesellschaft für Psychosomatische Medizin und Psychotherapie, Deutsche Gesellschaft für Ernährungsmedizin (2010c) ► literature 5.1

Wimmelmann CL, Dela F, Mortensen EL (2014a) Psychological predictors of mental health and health-related quality of life after bariatric surgery: a review of the recent research. Obes Res Clin Pract 8:e314–e324

Wimmelmann CL, Dela F, Mortensen EL (2014b) Psychological predictors of weight loss after bariatric surgery: a review of the recent research. Obes Res Clin Pract 8:e299–e313

5.4

Deutsche Adipositas-Gesellschaft, Deutsche Diabetes Gesellschaft, Deutsche Gesellschaft für Ernährung, deutsche Gesellschaft für Ernährungsmedizin (2014c) ► literature 5.1

Hüttl TP (2014) Adipositaschirurgie – Indikation, Operationsverfahren und Erfolgsaussichten. Klinikarzt 43:198–204

Runkel N, Colombo-Benkmann M, Hüttl TP et al (2011) Bariatric surgery. Dtsch Arztebl Int 108:341–346

5.5

Hüttl PE (2007) Aufklärung und Einwilligung. In: Heberer J (Hrsg) Recht im OP. MWV Medizinisch Wissenschaftliche Verlagsgesellschaft, Berlin, S 29–54

Hüttl PE, Hüttl TP (2010) Rechtsfragen der Adipositas Chirurgie. Der Chirurg BDC 9:485–492

Operation Preparation in Bariatric Surgery

J. Mall

Contents

© Springer-Verlag GmbH Germany, part of Springer Nature 2022
J. Ordemann, U. Elbelt (eds.), *Obesity and Metabolic Surgery*,
https://doi.org/10.1007/978-3-662-63227-7_6

6.1 Operating Room

Bariatric operations must take place in specially equipped operating theatres. In principle, a sufficiently large room with extra-wide operating tables or lafettes with sufficient load capacity of the operating column and sufficient space for several instrument tables of the instrumenting OR nursing staff is required. Movable monitors for laparoscopy, like laparoscopic instruments, are now standard equipment in most operating theatres. An additional monitor for anaesthesia is helpful. In many operating theatres, documentation of the operation on a hard disk (AIDA documentation system) has been established. This can provide valuable information, especially in the case of postoperative complications, for exact planning of the revision operation or for the tactical procedure of the treatment. Access to diagnostic image material in digital form is particularly helpful for redo operations in the operating room. Anaesthesiological aids such as extra-wide blood pressure cuffs, extra-wide armrests, positioning material for widening the operating table, sufficient padding material and video laryngoscopic instruments for managing difficult airways during intubation must also be available.

6.2 Instruments

Long laparoscopic instruments as well as conventional instruments of sufficient size must be kept in stock, although not necessary for every bariatric operation. Special laparoscopic hook systems (cook hooks, blue snake retractors, disposable laparoscopic retractors) must also always be available. Even if extra-long trocars are not required for every bariatric operation, they are often necessary, especially in cases with a BMI > 60 kg/m^2 and very obese abdominal walls. Monopolar and bipolar laparoscopic coagulation options are a matter of course. In addition, modern vascular sealing systems (Harmonic ace, LigaSure atlas clamp or similar) of sufficient length are required. Clip applicators as disposable or reusable devices are also often necessary to safely stop bleeding from the staple suture line or during preparation.

6.3 Positioning the Patient

Due to the higher weight of the patients, it can usually be assumed that an increased number of people will be required for positioning. However, in clinics that have a high frequency of operations on bariatric patients, this usually only applies to so-called super-obese patients, who can only get out of bed preoperatively with help. These patients have to be transported in special beds approved for this purpose into the operating theatre sluice. For the transfer process to the extra-wide surgical bed, 4–6 persons are usually required. For the remaining, preoperatively mobile patients, transfer to the operating table is usually possible without any problems with the help of a positioning nurse or an anaesthesia/surgical nurse. In some clinics, patients now walk into the operating room independently, wearing an operating shirt and disposable shoes, accompanied by an escort. In this case, however, the pre-medication with opiate-containing medication that is common in most anaesthesia departments must be omitted. This has the advantage of saving personnel resources; in addition, the patient is able to lie down on the operating table independently and notice possible positioning complications while still awake (e.g., pain when legs are spread too far apart, lumbar pain due to insufficient padding, etc.). Since almost all obese patients already show pathological changes in the large joints and the spinal column preoperatively, this procedure has proven itself in our own clinic in over 90% of patients and has almost eliminated the number of postoperative problems caused by incorrect positioning. For patients who are not independent, the exact padding of the back and buttocks with appropriate gel mats must be meticulously observed.

In Europe, the positioning is usually carried out in the so-called French technique (French Position) in the supine position with spread legs (■ Fig. 6.1).

In the positioning frequently performed in the USA, the patient also lies in a supine position, but the legs are not spread (■ Fig. 6.2).

For intubation, the patient is usually positioned in the so-called ramped position with elevation of the thorax by 30–40°. This can be achieved either by bending the table or by using

6

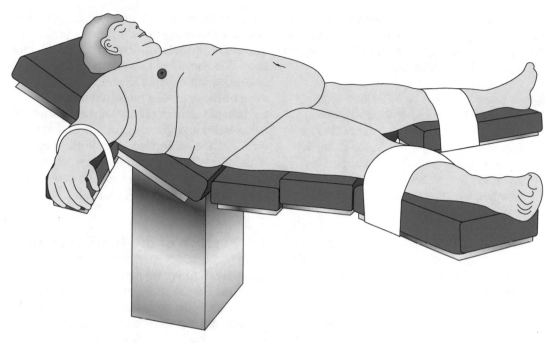

◨ **Fig. 6.1** French position

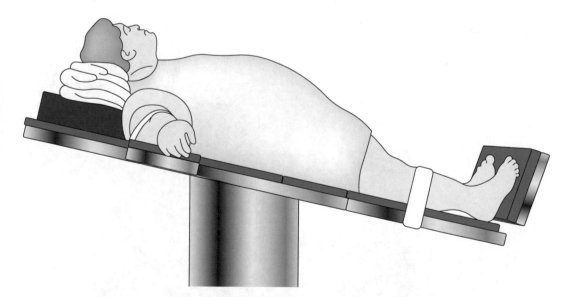

◨ **Fig. 6.2** American position

a positioning wedge cushion (Oxford cushion). In this way a reduction of the abdominal pressure on the diaphragm with a reduction of the dead space volume is achieved and thus better preoxygenation conditions before intubation.

According to the preference of the surgeon, the arms can usually both be transferred and fixed in 60–90° abduction on a padded arm splint or be positioned laterally.

A half-roll is placed under the back of the knee to relieve the legs. The heels are padded with gel pads. For very obese patients, it may be necessary to additionally attach a transverse board under the buttocks to prevent the patient from slipping during the operation. The legs are fixed, which is not always easy and without complications in very obese patients. Roller mats with a Velcro fastening have proven to be a good solution. They are simply wrapped around the entire leg and, if they fit well, prevent the patient from slipping even when the position is changed.

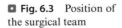 In general, it must be taken into account that, due to the highly variable physiognomy of obese patients and due to the fact that the position of the patient usually changes several times during the operation, good fixation without compromising the vessels or nerves of the patient's extremities is of enormous importance.

After successful intubation, a bladder catheter can be inserted. In most clinics with high operation frequency of bariatric patients this is avoided in the meantime due to an average operation time of ≤60 min. If the operations usually take longer than 90 min, catheterisation should be performed. After the usual skin disinfection and sterile covering of the patient, the table can be tilted into an anti-Trendelenburg position according to the surgeon's preference. The monitors for laparoscopy are placed on the head side above both shoulders of the patient at an adequate height. Depending on the equipment of the operating room, a third monitor in the field of vision of the anaesthetist has proven to be useful in order to ensure good communication of the entire team during the operation if the anaesthetist is required (e.g., change of position of the inserted stomach probe, leak test of the gastrojejunostomy, etc.).

6.4 Position of the Surgical Team

The operation is usually performed using the so-called French technique, in which the surgeon stands between the spread legs of the patient and the assistants are positioned on the left and/or right side (◘ Fig. 6.3). In most clinics, bariatric surgery is now performed in

◘ **Fig. 6.3** Position of the surgical team

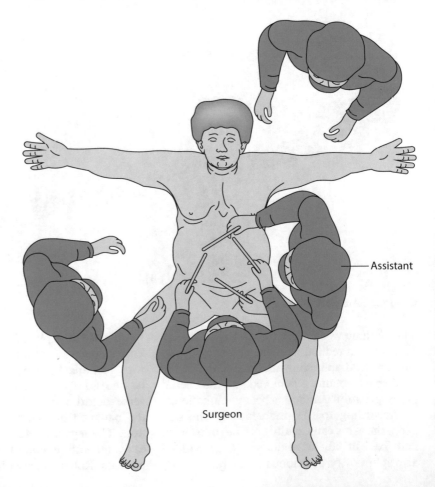

Assistant

Surgeon

pairs. However, for training purposes or in case of difficult anatomical conditions, a second assistant may be helpful and necessary. Some surgeons prefer the position on one side of the patient together with the assistant. In this case, the respective arm should be attached to the side. Otherwise, the arms are usually positioned out of alignment. Warming systems (Bair Hugger® warming units, blankets, etc.) can be placed up to the middle thorax and from the pelvis down to prevent the patient from cooling down during the operation.

6.5 Antibiotic Treatment

Perioperative antibiotic prophylaxis is standard procedure for bariatric surgery. Obesity is an independent risk factor for wound infections after any surgical procedure. As with other surgical procedures, perioperative prophylaxis should be administered 30–60 min before the incision. Due to obesity, changes in the pharmacokinetics and pharmacodynamics of the various substance classes must be taken into account during administration. There are no reliable scientific findings on the exact change in the dosage of most antibiotics in obese patients. Nevertheless, the following factors should be taken into account when selecting antibiotics:

- known drug allergies/intolerances,
- renal function restrictions,
- concomitant diseases with increased risk of infection,
- altered distribution volume of the drug (blood flow to the fatty tissue <5% of cardiac output, hydrophilicity/lipophilicity of the antibiotic),
- interaction with other pharmaceuticals,
- elimination of the antibiotic (hydrophilic antibiotics are excreted better).

The choice of antibiotic depends on the expected germ spectrum during the operation. As the stomach and small intestine are opened, a second or third generation cephalosporin is considered sufficient (e.g., cefazolin 2 g at BMI > 40 kg/m^2). It is recommended to repeat the administration if the operation lasts longer than 3–5 h. In case of a sufficient effect level, an earlier repetition is not reasonable from a pharmacological point of view and is not supported by scientific evidence. The addition of metronidazole or other antibiotics effective against anaerobic germs is not indicated.

An unsolved problem is the dosage of perioperative antibiotic prophylaxis in so-called super-obese patients with a BMI > 60 kg/m^2. In a comparative study by Edmiston et al. (2004) with a low number of cases, however, it was shown that in patients with a BMI > 60 kg/m^2 the effective concentration of 2 g cefazolin in the tissue was only 10%—compared to 48% in a patient with a BMI of 40 kg/m^2. However, there are currently no precise dosage recommendations for an increased dose adapted to an increase in BMI or total weight.

6.6 Anticoagulation

Obesity is a known risk factor for the occurrence of thromboembolic complications for a long time. The risk of postoperative thrombosis increases in severely obese patients not only due to the passage of perioperative immobilization, but especially due to the frequent presence of several risk factors associated with thrombosis in obese patients, such as arterial hypertension, hyperglycemia and varicosis. In addition, obese patients often have an increased coagulability, which in addition to platelet dysfunction leads to an overall increased tendency to thrombosis. According to studies by Buchwald et al. (2007), the incidence of pulmonary embolism after bariatric surgery is approximately 0.8%. For experienced bariatric surgeons, for whom technically induced postoperative complications are rare, thromboembolic complications thus represent a major risk factor for perioperative mortality. Statistically, the risk of thrombosis seems to be significantly increased with a BMI > 60 kg/m^2, especially if there is a simultaneous varicosis with chronic venous insufficiency. Therefore, some surgeons even recommend the prophylactic implantation of a cava-inferior umbrella for this group of patients preoperatively. However, the high rate of thrombosis after removal of the umbrella seems to outweigh the perioperative protective advantages, and thus, in the opinion of the author, their implantation is reserved for rare individual indications.

Optimal thromboembolic prophylaxis in obese patients prior to bariatric surgery has not yet been standardized. In particular, the dosage adjustments in super-obese patients—similar to the dosage of antibiotics in this patient group—have not been fully clarified. The operating surgeon is faced with the conflict between too low a dose of prophylaxis and an overdose with an increased risk of intra- and postoperative bleeding. In the case of a known thromboembolic complication, a coagulation physiological clarification of the patient is recommended. The concomitant medication (antiplatelet inhibitors, new direct oral anticoagulants (DOAC), Phenprocoumon) of the patient must be observed and, if necessary, discontinued or bridged.

According to data from the quality assurance study on surgical treatment of obesity from 2012, thromboembolism prophylaxis was performed in 96.8% of primary interventions in Germany. Low molecular weight heparins are administered most frequently. Newer, direct oral anticoagulants are currently not used. For none of the many available drugs have significant advantages over the others that been proven. Some authors stress the better controllability of unfractionated heparins compared to low-molecular-weight heparins, but this does not seem to

Table 6.1 Dosage scheme for thrombosis prophylaxis in bariatric operations

Patient weight (kg)	Thrombosis prophylaxis with	
	NMWH, for example enoxaparin	
<160 kg	40 mg s. c., 1-0-1/day	Alternatively 80 mg s. c., 1/day
>160 kg	60 mg s. c., 1-0-1/day	Alternatively 100–120 mg s. c., 1/day
	Fondaparinux	
	2.5 mg 1/day	

have a significant effect on the reduction of thromboembolism or the occurrence of bleeding intra- or postoperatively. There are no reliable findings that speak in favour of starting thrombosis prophylaxis preoperatively. The postoperative therapy can be continued weight-adapted, starting in the evening of the operation and continuing for 8 h a day until mobilisation. Enoxaparin is frequently administered—either as a single dose or in two doses, depending on the weight of the patient. Enoxaparin is the most frequently investigated low-molecular-weight heparin in the currently existing studies in obese patients. **Table 6.1** shows a possible schedule of administration.

To estimate and determine the dosage for very heavy body weight, the following formula should be used:

$$\text{Adjusted Dosage} = (\text{Total body weight in kg} - \text{Ideal weight}) \times 0.4 + \text{Ideal weight}$$

Fondaparinux may be administered in cases of known heparin-induced thrombocytopenia (HIT).

The significance of intraoperative intermittent sequential pneumatic compression therapy is currently not entirely clear. There are no studies that prove a reduction of

thromboembolic complications after bariatric surgery. The consensus is that patients should be mobilised as early as possible after surgery (in the recovery room or in the afternoon of the day of surgery). Intensive mobilisation is certainly also very relevant in the first few days following the operation in order to prevent thrombosis. Valid data on the duration of thrombosis prophylaxis with low molecular weight heparin are also not available. Recommendations in the literature vary between a few days and up to several months postoperatively.

6.7 Team Time Out

In recent years, checklists, which have been standard in the aviation industry for decades, have also been introduced in operating theatres to avoid confusion of procedures. Even though it is not necessarily possible to confuse an organ in bariatric surgery, it is still conceivable—especially in clinics with a high frequency of metabolic operations—that the planned procedure will be confused and a sleeve gastrectomy will be mistakenly inserted instead of a gastric bypass. Even though this risk is very small, it can be minimized even further by strictly adhering to a team timeout before the start of the operation using standardized checklists. A possible example of such a checklist is shown in ◻ Table 6.2. Usually, the retrieval of these checklists is embedded in a Standard Operating Procedure (SOP), in which preoperatively (when the patient is taken to the preparation room) a verification process of the patient identity and the planned intervention takes place between the professional groups involved in the treatment process.

◻ **Table 6.2** Team time-out surgery: example of a checklist before surgery

Theatre nurse asks the following questions loud and clear:	Answer:
All team members known?	All involved
Patient's name?	Anaesthetist
Patient's date of birth?	Anaesthetist
Known allergies?	Anaesthesia/ surgeon
Antibiotic administration necessary/successful?	Surgeon/ anaesthetist
Scheduled procedure?	Surgeon
Indication doctor?	Surgeon
Expected op duration/body side?	Surgeon
Pre-ops that affect this op?	Surgeon
Pacemaker/defibrillator?	Surgeon
Storage checked?	Surgeon/ anaesthetist
Blood loss expected?	Surgeon
Patient specific problems?	Anaesthetist
Neutral electrode applied?	Theatre nurse
Quick cut planned?	Surgeon
Equipment and sieves available/ sterile?	Theatre nurse
Identity and date of the image material?	Surgeon
Intraoperative documentation?	Surgeon

> **Practical Tip**
>
> Important for the success of a Team Time Out is the implementation in concrete organizational processes on the ward, in the recovery room and in the operating room.

Even in the case of necessary forensic assessments, a solid risk management can have a beneficial effect on affected hospital employees.

6.8 Structure of the Pneumoperitoneum

The formation of the pneumoperitoneum (capnoperitoneum) in obese patients is significantly more difficult than in non-adipose patients due to various factors. The different distribution of fat, the very variable distance from the xyphoid to the navel, abdominal pre-surgery as well as significant liver enlargement and a large distance from the skin to the peritoneum make access to the abdomen more difficult. While the discussion about the best and least risky access route to the site of the pneumoperitoneum is not conclusively clarified in the laparoscopy of non-adipose patients, additional problems arise in obese patients. Open access in obese patients usually means a larger incision to gain a clear view of the muscular abdominal wall and the underlying peritoneum. Consequently, after creation of the access and high-volume insufflation of CO_2, a higher gas loss during surgery must be expected. While the problem of gas loss rarely occurs when using the Verres needle, only a small volume of gas can be initially insufflated into the abdomen when using the Verres needle. The classic technique with the Verres needle with lifting of the abdominal wall and insertion of the needle is difficult to practice in the upper and middle abdomen in case of very obese abdominal wall, because the distance between skin and abdominal wall often even increases when lifting the fat layers and the actual muscular abdominal wall is not lifted at all. A puncture in the left upper abdomen below the left costal arch at the level of the midclavicular line (Palmer Point) is recommended. Here, adhesions are rarely found after previous median laparotomies, and experience shows that the abdominal wall is less thick. The position of the internal organs can vary considerably depending on the patient's position and increase the risk of organ injury. In the anti-Trendelenburg position, the often very large liver of the patient slips caudally and is thus exposed to an increased risk of injury. For this reason, the pneumoperitoneum should be established in a 180° supine position. If necessary, a preoperative ultrasound in the same position as in the operating room can provide valuable information on how to avoid injuries.

A third recommended option is the use of self-tapping trocars under camera view (so-called Visible Port). Here, after a small incision in the skin, the port is advanced under visual control with slight pressure and by means of rotary movements, and after passing through the peritoneum, gas insufflation begins under visual control. The advantage is the immediate control of trocar entry into the abdominal cavity and thus an expected minimization of the risk of injury to intra-abdominal organs. However, in the literature there are no statistically significant differences in the risk of injury to internal organs or vessels between the described procedures (Table 6.3).

The target pressure for bariatric surgery should be 15–20 mmHg. Note the diameter of the trocar through which gas insufflation is initiated: At least a 10–12 mm trocar should be used for permanent insufflation. Due to the high preload of the abdominal wall, the intraabdominal resting pressure of the obese patient is increased. The degree of relaxation of the patient and the shearing forces of the trocars can also have an influence on the continuity of the pneumoperitoneum, as can the use of the suction cup during insufflation. Some surgeons therefore prefer a high flow insufflator with a fixed pressure level and a high insufflation stroke in order to be able to quickly compensate pressure fluctuations caused by the influencing factors described above.

 Table 6.3 Advantages and disadvantages of different capnoperitoneum placement techniques

	Visible port	Verres needle	Open system
Preparation elaborate	No	No	Yes
Incision length	Small	Small	Large
Gas loss	No	No	Yes
Insufflation speed	High	Small	High
Security	High	Less	High
Relative contraindications	Abdominal pre-surgery	Abdominal pre-surgery	None

References

Buchwald H, Cowan GSM, Pories WJ (2007) Surgical management of obesity, 2nd edn. Saunders, Philadelphia, p 102

Edmiston CE, Krepel C, Kelly H, Larson J, Andris D, Hennen C, Nakeeb A, Wallace JR (2004) Perioperative antibiotic prophylaxis in the gastric bypass patient: do we achieve therapeutic levels? Surgery 136:738–747

Further Readings

Campello E, Zabeo E, Radu CM et al (2015) Hypercoagulability in overweight and obese subjects who are asymptomatic for thrombotic events. Thromb Haemost 113:85–96

Engeli S, Stroh C (2015) Adipositas und das Risiko für venöse Thrombosen und Embolien. Adipositas 9: 59–63

Holst AG, Jensen G, Prescott E (2010) Risk factors for venous thromboembolism: results from the Copenhagen City Heart Study. Circulation 121:1896–1903

Manjunath PP, Bearden DT (2007) Antimicrobial dosing considerations in obese adult patients. Pharmacotherapy 27:1081–1091

Morange PE, Alessi MC (2013) Thrombosis in central obesity and metabolic syndrome: mechanisms and epidemiology. Thromb Haemost 110:669–680

Roe JL, Fuentes JM, Mullins ME (2012) Underdosing of common antibiotics for obese patients in the ED. Am J Em Med 30:1212–1214

Utzolino S, Karcz K (2013) Thromboseprophylaxe in der bariatrischen Chirurgie. Phlebologie 42:71–76

Anaesthesiology for Bariatric Surgery

J. Birnbaum

Contents

© Springer-Verlag GmbH Germany, part of Springer Nature 2022
J. Ordemann, U. Elbelt (eds.), *Obesity and Metabolic Surgery*,
https://doi.org/10.1007/978-3-662-63227-7_7

The increasing awareness for anaesthesiological problems among patients with obesity or patients undergoing bariatric surgery is reflected in the increasing number of publications on this topic in recent years. In 2015, the Association of Anaesthetists of Great Britain and Ireland published exemplary guidelines on the perioperative management of obese surgical patients.

7.1 Pathophysiological Aspects

7.1.1 The Cardiovascular System

There is an increased absolute circulating blood volume in obese patients. However, the relative blood volume based on body weight is reduced. While normal patients have a blood volume of about 75 ml/kg total body weight, the relative blood volume in obese patients is reduced to about 45 ml/kg total body weight.

The cardiac output is often increased—mainly by increasing the stroke volume. Left ventricular hypertrophy is the result of pressure and volume loading. The systolic pumping function is partially restricted, as is the diastolic relaxation of the left ventricle. This can result in dilatation of the left atrium. Hence, compensation for circulatory stress, e.g., by increasing the stroke volume or the ejection fraction, is only possible to a limited extent.

The cardiovascular system as a whole is characterized by an increased sympathetic tone, and the autonomic nervous system may have impaired adrenergic reflexes. Hemodynamic instability during orthostasis or under stress is the result.

In addition to arterial hypertension obese patients often have arrhythmias, often due to AV node dysfunction and fat infiltration of the electrical conduction system of the heart. The consequence is an increased risk of atrial fibrillation or sudden cardiac death. Obesity is also associated with an increased incidence of prolongation of the QT interval. This is particularly important when using medications which can extend the QT interval (e.g., Ondansetron, Haldol etc.).

In obese patients, the prevalence of chronic ischemic heart disease and heart failure is increased. These are major risk factors for postoperative complications.

Since obesity is a prothrombotic condition, the risk of myocardial infarction, stroke and venous thromboembolism (VTE) is increased. VTE in medical history is a relevant risk factor. Adequate and sufficiently long postoperative thromboembolism prophylaxis is essential, as the hypercoagulable phase can exceed a duration of two weeks.

7.1.2 Airway

Obesity is very often associated with obstructive sleep apnea syndrome (OSAS). In obese patients and especially in OSAS patients, difficult intubation conditions are increasingly prevalent, caused by fat deposits in the tissue of the nasopharyngeal space. Although the frequency of difficult intubation conditions in obese patients has been overestimated in the past, it is still about 1%. Mask ventilation is difficult in about 10% of patients.

It should also be noted that OSAS itself is a risk factor for other comorbidities such as arterial hypertension, atrial fibrillation, cardiovascular disease, pulmonary hypertension or even depression.

7.1.3 Pulmonary System

The accumulation of fat can massively reduce compliance of the thoracic wall and the lungs themselves. The abdominal fat accumulation impairs diaphragmatic excursion and leads to a diaphragmatic elevation, especially in supine position, thus limiting the expansion of the lungs. The functional residual capacity (FRC), the expiratory reserve volume (ERV) and the total lung capacity (TLC) are reduced due to the mechanical influence of the fat masses. The necessary work of breathing is significantly increased, resulting in obesity hypoventilation syndrome (OHS). In addition, since oxygen consumption and CO_2 production are increased in obese patients, the oxygen saturation in the blood drops more rapidly during anaesthetic induction compared to healthy patients. Often a difficult mask ventilation can further aggravate the problem.

Depending on the position of the patient, this problem can be exacerbated intraoperatively (e.g., low head position, capnoperitoneum in laparoscopy, etc.). Especially the small airways can collapse under the pressure of the surrounding tissue. The lung volume at which the small airways collapse is called the closing capacity (CC). If the FRC impaired by the pathophysiological changes falls below the CC during machine ventilation, the small airways are repeatedly opened and closed. This mechanism can lead to ventilation-induced lung damage.

The resulting higher incidence of atelectasis in obese patients can lead to a more frequent drop in oxygen saturation in the postoperative phase.

Furthermore, an association between obesity with asthma has been described; this seems to be related to nocturnal gastroesophageal reflux. The incidence of bronchial asthma in obese patients is about twice as high as in normal weight patients.

7.1.4 Metabolism

Obesity is often associated with increased insulin resistance. Insufficient monitoring and control of glucose metabolism can increase perioperative morbidity. This is particularly relevant if a postoperative reduction in insulin demand occurs suddenly as a result of a gastric bypass. In this case, a rapid adjustment of antidiabetic medications and close blood glucose control are necessary.

7.1.5 Pharmacokinetics

Usually, drugs are dosed according to body weight. In obese patients, however, the proportion of body fat to total body weight is massively increased. Accordingly, the distribution of medication changes. Consequently,

different dosage scales must be applied for obese patients. Unfortunately, pharmacokinetic data for obese patients often only exist to a limited extent for many drugs, since obesity is often considered an exclusion criterion in clinical studies.

In principle, in obese patients, every available form of monitoring should be used, which, in addition to clinical evaluation, can provide further information on the effect of the substances applied (e.g. neuromonitoring, such as bispectral index BIS or patient state index PSI to measure the depth of anaesthesia, especially with total intravenous anaesthesia, and relaxometry to assess muscle relaxation).

An essential basis for the dosage of drugs is the body weight, even in obese patients. Starting from the total body weight, various other parameters are calculated.

Determination of Body Weight and Other Parameters

■ Total Body Weight (TBW)

In obese patients the TBW is composed of the lean body weight (LBW) and the fatty tissue. With increasing obesity, however, these two proportions do not increase in proportion to each other. The relative LBW proportion decreases with increasing TBW.

■ Body Mass Index (BMI)

The BMI is calculated from TBW divided by the height squared (see ► Chap. 1, ► Table 1.1):

$$BMI\left[kg/m^2\right] = \frac{TBW}{Body\ size^2}$$

To further classify extreme obesity, patients with a BMI > 50 are also referred to as super-obese and patients with a BMI > 60 as super-super-obese.

■ Body Surface Area (BSA)

Simplified, the body surface is calculated as follows:

$$BSA\left[m^2\right] = \frac{TBW \times Body\ size\ in\ cm}{3600} \times 0.5$$

■ **Ideal Body Weight (IBW)**

The ideal weight is based on a survey in the USA in which an attempt was made in the interest of life insurance companies to correlate an ideal body weight with maximum life expectancy.

The IBW can be calculated using an empirical formula:

$$Women: IBW = 45.4\,kg + 0.89 \\ \times (height\ in\ cm - 152.4)$$

$$Men: IBW = 49.9\,kg + 0.89 \\ \times (height\ in\ cm - 152.4)$$

With the ideal body weight, the body constitution, apart from the height, is not taken into account.

■ **Fat-Free Body Mass (Lean Body Weight, LBW)**

The fat-free body mass, also known as lean body mass, characterizes the body weight minus the total fat tissue.

The LBW can be calculated approximately using the following formulas:

$$Women: LBW = 1.07 \times TBW - 0.0148 \\ \times BMI \times TBW$$

$$Men: LBW = 1.1 \times TBW - 0.0128 \\ \times BMI \times TBW$$

The pharmacokinetics of the drugs used in obese patients, i.e. their distribution, binding, storage and elimination, is influenced by various factors. The proliferation of fatty tissue may significantly influence the distribution volume of drugs used under anaesthesia. This is particularly true for lipophilic substances, whereas the distribution of hydrophilic substances is only slightly influenced. Also, the increased total blood volume, the increased cardiac output and an altered plasma-protein binding play a relevant role. A significantly prolonged elimination half-life compared to normal weight patients can be the result.

In addition to the influences of obesity, the effects of concomitant diseases on pharmacokinetics must be taken into account. In particular, changes in hepatic or renal clearance play an important role. Depending on the stage of the disease, the clearance can be either reduced or increased. Therefore, the renal clearance should be determined in case of doubt.

Thus, in comparison to normal weight patients, both the patient-specific pathophysiological situation and its influence on the pharmacokinetics of the respective drug must be taken into account. In the following, the pharmacokinetic peculiarities of typical drugs used during anaesthesia in connection with obesity will be discussed.

Pharmacokinetic Characteristics of Important Substances

■ **Benzodiazepines**

As a result of the high lipophilicity of benzodiazepines, the distribution volume is increased due to the fat accumulation of these substances. Accordingly, the dose should be increased in proportion to the TBW. It should be noted, however, that in continuous infusions the dosage should be more in line with the IBW, since clearance is not affected (apart from liver or kidney dysfunction). If OSAS is present, a contraindication to benzodiazepines must be taken into account.

■ **Propofol**

Propofol is characterized by a high lipophilicity (fat emulsion). Due to its pharmacological properties, Propofol is well suited both as a substance for hypnotic induction and for maintaining anaesthesia in obese patients. After injection, Propofol rapidly crosses the blood-brain barrier (rapid onset). This leads to rapid redistribution in muscle and fat tissue. The distribution volume correlates well with TBW, and there is no relevant accumulation or prolongation of effect. Thus, the dosage of both induction and maintenance of anaesthesia can be oriented to the TBW.

■ **Thiopental**

The injection of thiopental also leads to a rapid onset of anaesthesia. After distribution in tissues with a high blood supply, there is a rapid redistribution, mainly in the muscles, but also in the fatty tissue. Due to the long elimination half-life (5–10 h), there is a risk of accumulation with repeated administration or even continuous infusion. The decrease of the plasma concentration is then mainly determined by the absorption into the fatty tissue and the hepatic elimination. The dosage in obese patients is based on the LBW.

▪ Etomidate

Up to now, there are insufficient data on the pharmacokinetics of etomidate in obese patients. Due to some side effects (reversible inhibition of steroid synthesis at higher doses, myoclonia, increased incidence of postoperative nausea and vomiting, injection pain) the use of etomidate is often limited to the induction of anaesthesia in haemodynamically unstable patients. This should not be handled differently in obese patients. Because of the similarity to thiopental, it seems to make sense to dose etomidate according to the LBW.

▪ Muscle Relaxants

The effect of hydrophilic muscle relaxants is not significantly affected by the presence of obesity.

An advantage of using succinylcholine is the fast onset time in connection with the often rapid oxygen desaturation in obese patients. Since the activity of plasma cholinesterase is often increased in highly obese patients, a dosage corresponding to the TBW seems to be reasonable. In obese patients the incidence of postoperative muscle pain after administration of succinylcholine is low.

Rocuronium as a non-depolarising muscle relaxant is also well suited for obese patients due to its relatively fast onset time. The substance is only slightly lipophilic. In extremely obese patients, however, rocuronium may have a significant prolongation of action when dosed according to TBW. To avoid a prolongation of the effect, the dosage should be according to IBW. As an antagonist for rocuronuim, sugammadex can be used to maintain good muscle relaxation until the end of surgery, if necessary, and to achieve rapid recovery from neuomuscular blockade. The elimination of sugammadex (as a

complex with rocuronium) depends on kidney function. The administration of sugammadex is contraindicated in cases of relevant impairment of renal function. To date, there are insufficient data on pharmacokinetics in obese patients.

Cis-atracurium is also well suited for use in obesity because of the Hoffmann elimination (organ-independent and pH and temperature-dependent decay). The duration of action can be prolonged compared to normal weight patients when dosed according to both TBW and IBW. Therefore, a dosage according to IBW is recommended.

In obese patients, relaxometry should always be used because of the various factors influencing the duration of neuromuscular blockade.

> **Practical Tip**
>
> Consistent use of relaxometry and individual muscle relaxation adapted to clinical requirements can reduce the risk of postoperative relaxant overhang and limit the need for antagonization of the neuromuscular blockade to exceptional cases.

▪ Inhalation Anaesthetics

The pharmacokinetics of volatile anaesthetics is essentially characterized by their lipophilicity. Due to the lower lipophilicity of sevoflurane and desflurane compared to isoflurane, these substances are more suitable for obese patients, because a faster recovery from anaesthesia is achieved. With desflurane there do not seem to be any relevant differences between obese and non-obese patients. In highly obese patients, the uptake and elimination of sevoflurane seems to be faster compared to isoflurane. In these severely overweight patients, desflurane and sevoflurane do not differ relevantly in their kinetics of induction and recovery. More lipophilic volatile anaesthetics accumulate in the fatty tissue after long (more than 2–4 h) anaesthesia and thus require a longer recovery time. After prolonged inhalation anaesthesia, the recovery phase after desflurane seems to be somewhat more favourable in obese patients than after sevoflurane in this respect.

■ **Opioids**

The clinically common synthetic opioids are characterized by their strong lipophilicity.

Fentanyl should be dosed according to LBW. As with sufentanil, which is also highly lipophilic, the initial clearance of fentanyl is higher in obese patients than in normal weight patients, so the initial plasma levels are lower. However, the dosage should be based on the LBW. These considerations can also be applied to sufentanil.

After application, remifentanil is rapidly hydrolyzed by esterases and thus converted into inactive substances. The pharmacokinetic parameters correlate well with the IBW. Remifentanil is characterised by a short onset time, the high clearance reduces the risk of postoperative prolongation.

❗ Especially in bariatric patients, the risk of a postoperative opioid overhang must be taken into account under any circumstances! Opioids in particular must be titrated individually according to their effect!

■ **Local Anaesthetics**

For various reasons, regional anaesthesiological techniques are also and especially suitable for use in obese patients. For example, the intra- and postoperative need for opioids is reduced, thus the opioid-related side effects can also be reduced. Here, especially the postoperative opioid-induced respiratory depression plays an important role.

When selecting the local anaesthetic, the same indications and contraindications must be taken into account in obese patients as in non-adipose patients. The systemic distribution with potential side effects is primarily dependent on the injection site; obesity does not seem to play a significant role here.

In connection with pharmacokinetics in obesity, data is available for lidocaine. Accordingly, lidocaine should be dosed according to TBW. For prilocaine and ropivacaine, the data are not sufficient in obese patients. The maximum dosages play a role particularly in wound infiltrations. In the case of peripheral nerve blocks, a reduction in the amount of local anaesthetic required can be achieved, particularly with the use of ultrasound.

It should also be noted that in the case of epidural and intrathecal application of local anaesthetics (epidural or spinal anaesthesia), lower amounts of local anaesthetic are required in obese patients than in normal weight patients in order to achieve the same level of blockage. The smaller cerebrospinal fluid volume compared to normal weight patients probably plays a role in the spread of spinal anaesthesia.

7.2 Organisational Aspects

In connection with the clinical treatment of extremely obese patients, organisational problems can easily arise in addition to medical ones. Of course, a hospital equipped for bariatric interventions must have identified and solved these potential problems in advance. Of concern is, for example, the provision of suitable beds and operating tables with sufficient load-bearing capacity or the appropriate equipment of the patient rooms (seating furniture, toilet seats, etc.). However, other hospitals can also be confronted with extremely obese patients at any time as part of emergency care.

7.2.1 Personnel

The anaesthesiological care of obese patients should in principle be entrusted to experienced anaesthesiological staff. For this purpose, it is helpful if a person responsible for these patients is appointed in every hospital. This is also laid down, for example, in the guidelines of the Association of Anaesthetists of Great Britain and Ireland on the perioperative management of obese surgical patients.

❗ In connection with airway management in obese patients, complications are more common if the anaesthesiological staff is inexperienced.

7.2.2 Technical Equipment

In addition to the basic technical requirements for the care of morbidly obese patients (e.g. operating tables are often designed for a body weight of up to 150 kg), the use of some technical aids is necessary or strongly recommended for anaesthesiological care.

Blood Pressure Measurement

The correct application of an upper arm blood pressure cuff often causes problems for morbidly obese patients. Suitable, oversized cuffs must be kept in stock in various sizes. The indication for an invasive blood pressure measurement should be generously set for both blood pressure measurement and arterial blood gas analysis.

Storage Material

To induce anaesthesia, the patient can be positioned with the upper body elevated or in the so-called ramp position (placing a large wedge cushion under the upper body). The tragus of the ear is at the level of the sternum (◘ Fig. 7.1). The aim is to improve lung mechanics and, consecutively, to improve oxygenation and ventilation and reduce the risk of regurgitation and aspiration.

Ultrasound

Especially for obese patients, ultrasound is a versatile tool. This refers, for example, to the performance of regional anaesthesia procedures both peripherally and near the spinal cord.

Establishing vascular access using ultrasound is often much easier than puncturing according to anatomical landmarks. In addition, the risk of puncture-related complications can be significantly reduced. Ultrasound is suitable for central as well as arterial and peripheral access. In particular, it should be used as standard when establishing central venous access.

Under difficult auscultation conditions after intubation, ultrasound can also be used to verify the diaphragm and the pleura movements to ensure an equal ventilation of both lungs (sliding sign).

7.3 Pre-medication Rounds

The pre-medication visit is essential for the evaluation of patients and should be conducted by a physician experienced with these patients. Ideally, a written standard (Standard Operating Procedure, SOP) exists for this purpose in a facility where bariatric procedures are performed more frequently.

The time for the pre-medication visit should be chosen sufficiently early so that there is enough time before the procedure to organize further individual preoperative diagnostics and, if necessary, therapy. These are essentially based on the comorbidities.

Even if it seems self-evident, it should be ensured that the exact weight, height and BMI are recorded (measured and weighed!) and documented as part of the preparation of the patient!

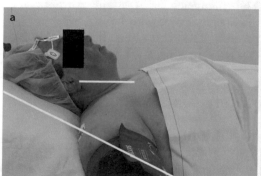 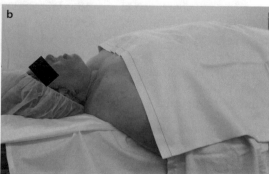

◘ **Fig. 7.1** **a** Ramp position: Patient positioning on a wedge cushion with raised upper body (see text). **b** Flat positioning of the patient after intubation. Here the difference to the ramp position is particularly clear

Practical Tip

The surgical plan should include patient weight and BMI!

Some specific aspects will be discussed below:

7.3.1 Pre-medication Consultation

When patients decide to undergo bariatric surgery because of high obesity, the level of suffering is often high. At the time of the anaesthesiological presentation, they practically always have a detailed psychological evaluation and, if necessary, intervention behind them. A high proportion of up to 35% of patients report clinically relevant symptoms of depression at the time of surgical evaluation. Accordingly, the empathy of the anaesthetist during the pre-medication consultation is of great importance.

7.3.2 Comorbidities

The Edmonton Obesity Staging System (EOSS) was developed to better classify the degree of pathophysiological changes. Patients are classified into a staging system between stage 0 (no signs of obesity-associated risk factors, no physical or psychological symptoms, no functional limitations) and stage 4 (severe obesity-associated comorbidities or severely impairing psychological symptoms or severe functional limitations). This classification is helpful to better assess perioperative risk, but it does not replace careful anaesthesiological evaluation. A more detailed description of this staging system is given in ▶ Sect. 5.1.

The relevance of some of the concomitant diseases will be explained in more detail here in connection with the pre-medication rounds and the preoperative evaluation of patients.

Respiratory System

The preoperative evaluation of the respiratory system depends on the severity of the obesity and the clinical symptoms. An X-ray of the thorax as initial findings, a pulmonary func-

tion test and an arterial blood gas analysis may be indicated.

During the pre-medication visit, patients should be examined for signs of a difficult airway (e.g., Mallampati score). Clinical experience shows that the majority of bariatric patients do not experience intubation problems. This requires careful evaluation of the airway, optimal patient positioning and the provision of additional aids for managing the difficult airway (video laryngoscope, etc.).

The systematic screening of obese patients for signs of obstructive sleep apnea syndrome (OSAS) is important. Indications of an existing OSAS can be excessive daytime sleepiness (evaluation by means of the Epworth Sleepiness Scale, ESS) or snoring and observed breathing stops. The diagnosis is made by overnight polysomnography in the sleep laboratory. A nocturnal, also ambulant polygraph can give first indications. The device can also be applied relatively easily by the patient himself and provides immediately evaluable results.

For patients with diagnosed OSAS, a longer-term preoperative therapy, usually nocturnal CPAP therapy, would be the optimal approach. In case of doubt, patients should be treated as if they had OSAS (e.g., postoperative intensive care, oxygen supplementation, CPAP therapy).

Smoking is also a risk factor for bariatric patients. Smoking abstention for 8 weeks preoperatively would be optimal. This should be initiated during the evaluation phase for a bariatric intervention.

Cardiovascular System

The frequency of relevant cardiovascular diseases increases with body weight in obese patients. The correlations have already been described in ▶ Sect. 7.1.1.

7.4 Preparation of the Anaesthesia

7.4.1 Monitoring

In principle, intraoperative monitoring does not differ from that of normal weight patients. The necessity of extended monitoring depends on the concomitant diseases. An exception is the measurement of arterial blood pressure. Automatic, non-invasive oscillotonometric blood pressure measurement using upper arm cuffs often reaches its limits due to extreme obesity and the resulting circumferences of the extremities. Therefore, the indication for invasive arterial blood pressure measurement should be given generously.

The following monitoring should be used as standard for highly obese patients:

- ECG monitor
- Pulse oximetry
- Arterial blood pressure measurement (non-invasive or invasive)
- Relaxometry
- Respiratory gas analysis
- Temperature probe
- Monitoring of the depth of anaesthesia (e.g., SEDLine, BIS)

7.4.2 Vascular Accesses

Creating a venous vascular access can be difficult in extremely obese patients. In most cases, however, a sufficiently large vein can be punctured conventionally or with the aid of ultrasound. This is often successful both on the forearm and especially in the crook of the arm (◘ Fig. 7.2). In the example shown in this figure, frustrating puncture attempts on the back of the hand were preceded, but with the help of ultrasound it was then very easy to puncture a relatively large vein in the crook of the elbow.

As a last resort, central venous catheter placement remains. From a surgical point of view, a central venous catheter is usually not indicated. In principle, the indication for a central venous catheter should be strictly defined for highly obese patients. Poor peripheral venous conditions should only be an indication for this if no peripheral venous accesses can be established using ultrasound.

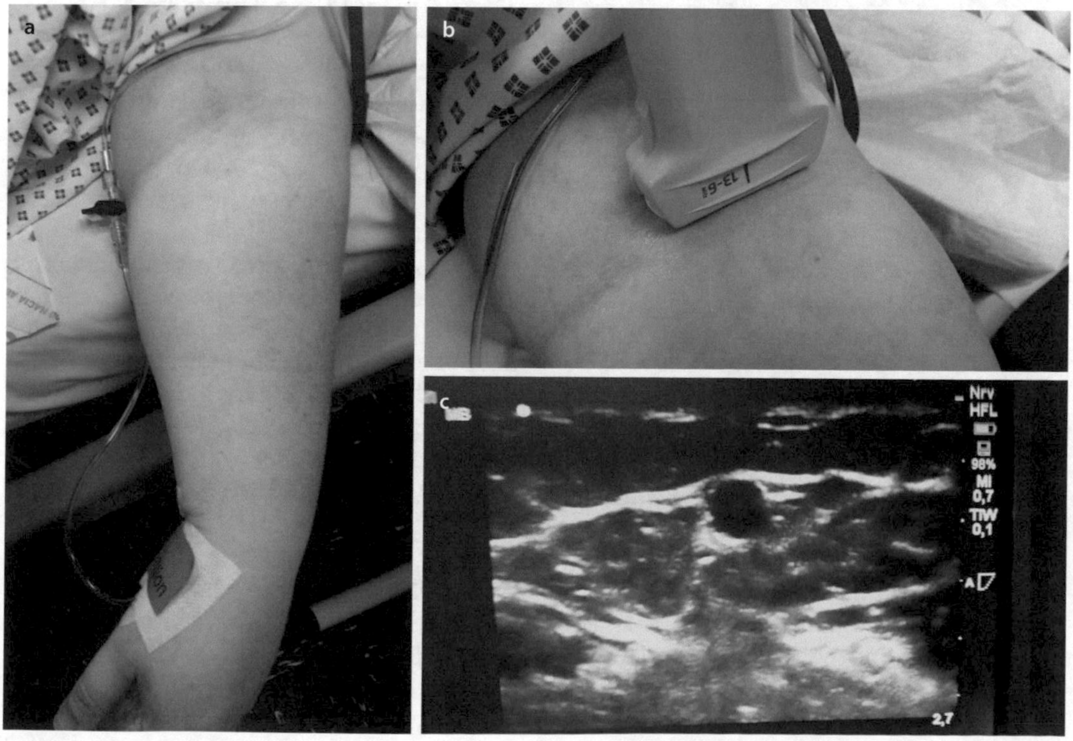

◘ **Fig. 7.2** Venous vascular access may be possible in an obese patient. **a** Venous condition on the forearm. **b** Placing the ultrasound probe in the crook of the arm. **c** Ultrasound image with relatively large vein, which can be easily punctured under ultrasound control approx. 7 mm below the skin surface

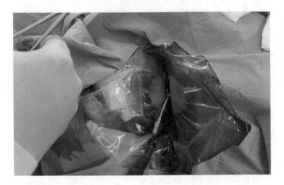

☐ Fig. 7.3 Central venous catheter in the right internal jugular vein in an obese patient

In addition to the already often difficult anatomical conditions at the neck in the region of the internal jugular vein as the puncture site of choice with consecutive risks of failure of puncture attempts and corresponding complications (☐ Fig. 7.3), a prothrombotic situation often prevails in these patients. This can result in thrombosis in the punctured veins.

> **Practical Tip**
>
> The puncture of a central vein should, as with all patients, generally be performed under direct ultrasound guidance!

The puncture for arterial access can also be performed under direct ultrasound guidance. Here too, sonography can help to shorten the puncture time and avoid complications (e.g. haematomas, nerve lesions).

7.4.3 Selection of Anaesthetics

The pharmacological principles and particularities in obese patients have already been explained in ▶ Sect. 7.1.5.

When selecting anaesthetics, as with all patients, the corresponding indications, contraindications and concomitant diseases of the patients are taken into account. Thus, relatively short-acting and easily controllable substances are available to avoid postoperative overhang. The dosage instructions relevant for obese patients must be observed.

Opioids in particular should be dosed carefully and sparingly to minimise opioid-related side effects. A combination of NSAIDs and local wound infiltration of local anaesthetics is helpful here.

7.5 Induction and Maintenance of Anaesthesia

7.5.1 Preoxygenation

Positioning the patient in the ramp position already explained in ▶ Sect. 7.2.2, in an approximately 30° anti-Trendelenburg position, PEEP (positive end-expiratory pressure) application for approximately 5 min or nasal intermittent ventilation with positive pressure (NIPPV) prior to initiation can extend the safe apnea time until intubation. Elevation of the upper body can reduce intra-abdominal pressure and decrease the risk of reflux.

7.5.2 Anaesthetic Induction

Although even highly obese patients can usually be intubated without any problems, alternative means of securing the airway should be kept available (e.g., video laryngoscope, etc.) due to the increased incidence of difficult intubations.

The necessity of rapid sequence induction (RSI) in obese patients was often discussed. In fact, the risk of aspiration seems to be quite low in these patients. The indication for a classic RSI should therefore be individualized and not routinely established. The commonly used induction anaesthetics are used in adapted dosages (▶ Sect. 7.1.5).

7.5.3 Maintenance of Anaesthesia

Both the usual volatile and intravenous anaesthetics are suitable for maintaining anaesthesia (sevoflurane, desflurane, propofol). The depth of anaesthesia is controlled according to clinical aspects and by neuromonitoring.

It is possible that substances such as the alpha-2 agonists, clonidine and dexmedetomidine, can reduce the need for anaesthetics and analgesics intra- and postoperatively. Also, completely opioid-free regimens (propofol, ketamine and dexmedetomidine) have recently been the subject of clinical research in bariatric surgery. This showed a significant reduction of nausea and vomiting in the perioperative phase (PONV) compared to a regime with volatile anaesthetics and opioids.

Adequate ventilation can be a challenge, especially during laparoscopic procedures. Although recruitment manoeuvres and ventilation with a PEEP of up to 1 mmHg can prevent atelectasis and improve intraoperative oxygenation, high ventilation pressures combined with increased intra-abdominal pressure and anti-Trendelenburg positioning have a negative impact on cardiac output and may induce barotrauma of the lung.

Patients are usually extubated in the operating room immediately after the procedure.

7.6 Postoperative Phase

There are no special recommendations with a sufficient level of evidence for the postoperative care of bariatric patients. So, one must refer mainly to the recommendations for obese patients.

Post-operative monitoring and therapy are based on the specifics of the individual patient and his or her secondary diseases, the course of the intervention and the organisational characteristics of the respective institution.

Ensuring adequate oxygenation plays an important role. Patients with OSAS should use their CPAP device for night sleep in any case. CPAP or non-invasive ventilation (NIPPV) can improve oxygenation and lung function. The impact of these measures on patient outcome remains the subject of clinical research. The necessity of intensive care monitoring and therapy should be assessed in appreciation of all accompanying circumstances (type and severity of secondary diseases, pain therapy, etc.).

The postoperative pain therapy should be carried out in an opioid-saving manner if possible. NSAIDs play an essential role here. It is recommended to use systemic and spinal cord opioids with restraint. However, sufficient data for this recommendation are also not yet available. As with all patients who are administered opioids, monitoring of the degree of sedation is necessary.

Regional anaesthesiological procedures (epidural anaesthesia, rectus sheath block, transversus-abdominis-plane block, etc.) can lead to improved pain control and have an opioid-saving effect.

As part of a fast-track strategy, it is advisable to mobilize patients as early as possible and to offer oral fluid already in the recovery room.

Further Readings

Andersen LP, Werner MU, Rosenberg J, Gögenur I (2014) Analgesic treatment in laparoscopic gastric bypass surgery: a systematic review of randomized trials. Obes Surg 24:462–470

Donohoe CL, Feeney C, Carey MF, Reynolds JV (2011) Perioperative evaluation of the obese patient. J Clin Anesth 23:575–586

Fleisher LA, Fleischmann KE, Auerbach AD et al (2014) American College of Cardiology; American Heart Association. 2014 ACC/AHA guideline on perioperative cardiovascular evaluation and management of patients undergoing noncardiac surgery: a report of the American College of Cardiology/American Heart Association Task Force on practice guidelines. J Am Coll Cardiol 64:e77–e137

Harbut P, Gozdzik W, Stjernfält E, Marsk R, Hesselvik JF (2014) Continuous positive airway pressure/pressure support pre-oxygenation of morbidly obese patients. Acta Anaesthesiol Scand 58:675–680

Huschak G, Busch T, Kaisers UX (2013) Obesity in anesthesia and intensive care. Best Pract Res Clin Endocrinol Metab 27:247–260

Jacobsen HJ, Bergland A, Raeder J, Gislason HG (2012) High-volume bariatric surgery in a single center: safety, quality, cost-efficacy and teaching aspects in 2000 consecutive cases. Obes Surg 22:158–166

Kuk JL, Ardern CI, Church TS et al (2011) Edmonton Obesity Staging System: association with weight history and mortality risk. Appl Physiol Nutr Metab 36:570–576

Lewandowski K, Lewandowski M (2011) Intensive care in the obese. Best Pract Res Clin Anaesthesiol 25:95–108

Leykin Y, Miotto L, Pellis T (2011) Pharmacokinetic considerations in the obese. Best Pract Res Clin Anaesthesiol 25:27–36

Lindauer B, Steurer MP, Müller MK, Dullenkopf A (2014) Anesthetic management of patients undergoing bariatric surgery: two year experience in a single institution in Switzerland. BMC Anesthesiol 14:125

Nightingale CE, Margarson MP, Shearer E et al (2015) Peri-operative management of the obese surgical patient 2015: Association of Anaesthetists of Great Britain and Ireland Society for Obesity and Bariatric Anaesthesia. Anaesthesia 70:859–876

Reusz G, Csomos A (2015) The role of ultrasound guidance for vascular access. Curr Opin Anaesthesiol 28:710–716

Schug SA, Raymann A (2011) Postoperative pain management of the obese patient. Best Pract Res Clin Anaesthesiol 25:73–81

Schumann R (2011) Anaesthesia for bariatric surgery. Best Pract Res Clin Anaesthesiol 25:83–93

Sharma AM, Kushner RF (2009) A proposed clinical staging system for obesity. Int J Obes 33:289–295

Weingarten TN, Hawkins NM, Beam WB et al (2015) Factors associated with prolonged anesthesia recovery following laparoscopic bariatric surgery: a retrospective analysis. Obes Surg 25:1024–1030

Ziemann-Gimmel P, Goldfarb AA, Koppman J, Marema RT (2014) Opioid-free total intravenous anaesthesia reduces postoperative nausea and vomiting in bariatric surgery beyond triple prophylaxis. Br J Anaesth 112:906–911

7

Laparoscopic, Adjustable Gastric Banding

H. Köhler

Contents

© Springer-Verlag GmbH Germany, part of Springer Nature 2022
J. Ordemann, U. Elbelt (eds.), *Obesity and Metabolic Surgery*,
https://doi.org/10.1007/978-3-662-63227-7_8

8.1 Trocar Placement

The storage and the build-up of the pneumoperitoneum are carried out as described in ▶ Chap. 6. As in most bariatric surgeries, the first trocar of 10 is placed paramedianally about 15 cm below the xiphoid on the left side. After the pneumoperitoneum has been built up, the abdomen is viewed from all sides. The patient is then positioned in the anti-Trendelenburg position for the rest of the operation. Then a 5-piece trocar is inserted into the right lateral upper abdomen, which should be done under visual control. The liver retractor is then inserted via this trocar and the left flap is lifted. If the position is correct, the liver retractor is then attached to a fixed holding system.

> ❶ It is now essential to prevent the patient from slipping, so that liver injuries caused by the retractor cannot occur.

For uncomplicated operations two additional working trocars are sufficient. The stitch direction during placement is extremely important, because in the case of thick abdominal walls, mobility is very limited afterwards.

A 5 trocar is placed in the right upper abdomen between the anterior axillary line and the midclavicular line at least 5 cm below the costal arch and runs diagonally in a craniomedial direction towards the base of the right diaphragm. The angulation instrument, e.g., the so-called goldfinger, is later inserted via this trocar. This should rise as steeply as possible from the caudal to the angle of His in order to achieve a 45° placement of the ligament.

A trocar of 10 is placed in the left upper abdomen between the anterior axillary line and the midclavicular line just below the costal arch. The ligament is later inserted via this access, even after the incision has been widened, and the port is placed. The incision is therefore made paracostally. The direction of the incision also runs craniomedially towards the cardia. Alternatively, a 15-piece trocar can be selected here for band insertion (❏ Fig. 8.2).

Additional 5-person trocars can be added optionally in case of difficult situs, e.g. left or right between the optical and working trocar.

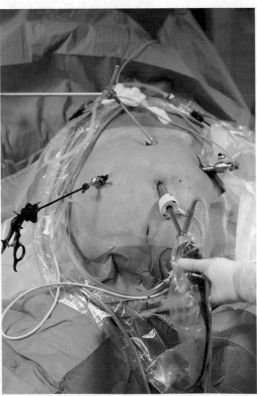

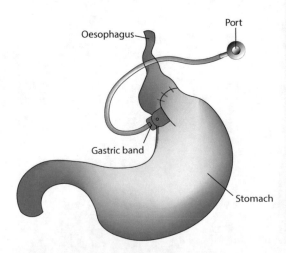

❏ **Fig. 8.1** Laparoscopic gastric band

❏ **Fig. 8.2** Trocar placement

8

8.2 Dissection

The anatomical landmarks are identified before the dissection begins. The lobus caudatus shines through the pars flaccida of the small net. The gastroesophageal junction is identified by advancement of a 36 Ch gastric tube. By tensing the fundus tip caudally, the angle of His and the upper spleen pole and the distal esophagus are shown from the left side.

The dissection begins at the angle of His so that a possible hiatal hernia can be detected. Larger hernias must be reduced and the hiatus closed to prevent dislocation of the ligament into the mediastinum. The peritoneal covering is opened over 2 cm between the angle of His and the diaphragm and the left diaphragm is shown. Lateral to the preparation the left arteria phrenica inferior, which has to be protected.

Subsequently, the avascular area of the pars flaccida of the small mesh is split with dissecting scissors or by diathermy and the base of the right diaphragm is shown. The gastroesophageal junction is splinted through a 36 Ch gastric tube and is bluntly luxated ventrally through the left approach with open grasping forceps. Now the peritoneal cover at the base of the right diaphragm can be dissected and spread from the right side with grasping forceps. The preparation is performed above the left gastric vessels and above the bursa omentalis. The instrument slides without resistance on the diaphragm through the retrocardial fat in a left-cranial direction towards the left diaphragmatic leg. The oesophagus, which is splinted ventrally through the stomach tube, can be palpated.

The grasping forceps are now exchanged for an angulating instrument, which is inserted into the traced retrogastric tunnel in a stretched position. With the right hand, the tip of the fundus is luxated caudally and the left diaphragm is shown. The instrument is then angulated until the tip shimmers through under the remaining tissue (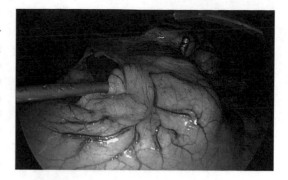 Fig. 8.3). The tissue can be bluntly removed with a preparation swab or a dissector. If the instrument is used to charge the stomach wall, the tip will

Fig. 8.3   Placement of the angulation instrument

not shine through. The same applies if the instrument enters the mediastinum behind the left diaphragm.

All in all, the entire preparation should be done very sparingly in order to create a good dorsal fixation for the band later on. If the instrument is correctly placed retroesophageally, the stomach tube should be pushed back and forth into the esophagus by the anaesthetist to verify correct positioning. This allows the correct position to be checked easily.

8.3 Placement of Gastric Band

The band can either be passed directly through the abdominal wall after removal of the 10 mm trocar in the left upper abdomen and digital expansion of the canal, or a 15 mm trocar is selected. After a tightness test and complete deflation, the band is moistened, grasped with atraumatic grasping forceps at the tip of the closure flap and stretched along the forceps shaft so that the balloon lies protected against the shaft. Now the tape is carefully guided into the abdominal cavity and the port tube is pushed in. A short-term loss of gas is usually not a problem. A grasping forceps is now inserted via the right working trocar, the loop on the gastric band closure is grasped and hooked into the groove of the angulated device. An additional 5-piece trocar should be of assistance during the first operations.

Before the band is now gently pulled through the retrogastric tunnel, it is impor-

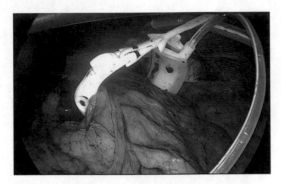

Fig. 8.4 Gastric band placed before closure and before application of fixation sutures

8

tant to stretch the angulated instrument again to avoid dorsal esophageal injuries. The tape should be pulled through slowly so that the tissue can yield without injury (Fig. 8.4). After pulling through, the angulation instrument is exchanged for an atraumatic grasping forceps and the correct position is checked again by pulling back the stomach tube and pushing it forward again. Before the band is closed ventrally, the stomach tube should be pulled back again. The different manufacturers offer different closures. The surgeon must be familiar with the closure technique of the implanted gastric band.

The pouch should be as small as possible (with a volume of approximately 15 ml), otherwise the risk of slipping and pouch dilatation increases.

Practical Tip

Using a calibration balloon on the stomach tube can be helpful to achieve a defined pouch size.

The closed gastric band should not be placed too tightly and should be able to be loosely passed under with an instrument. The closure and port tube are placed on the small-curvature side in order to have sufficient distance to the spleen in case of a later explantation or ligament correction.

8.4 Fixing the Gastric Band and Port

After placement of the tape, up to 4 serous sutures are applied from the fundus to the pouch to prevent the tape from slipping distally (Fig. 8.5). Especially on the left lateral side the fundus has to be fixed. Therefore, the fundus is rather pulled over the ligament from the left lateral to medial than from caudal to cranial. In this way a 45° positioning of the implant is achieved.

If a tension-free attachment of the fundus to the pouch cannot be achieved, the fundus tip can alternatively be fixed to the left cranial diaphragm. In addition, the medial fundus can be guided and fixed to the right diaphragmatic leg via the implant to achieve a secure attachment. Basically, a tension-free cuff must be constructed. The sutures must be applied with non-resorbable sutures. When piercing the stomach wall, a strictly seromuscular course of the sutures must be ensured.

> In case of a completely transmural course with perforation of the mucosa, germ transfer along the suture with implant infection and/or migration occurs.

When pricking the pouch wall with a curved needle, there is a risk of implant injury with the back of the needle. The band must be pressed securely caudally with grasping for-

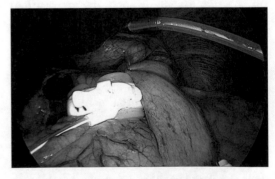

Fig. 8.5 Closed gastric band after application of the serous sutures

ceps. When knotting, ensure a secure serous contact of the stomach walls. If this results in an "air knot", after filling the band the thread can cut the balloon and lead to a leakage.

Fixation of the ventral aspect of the fundus wall can significantly reduce the risk of slipping, but not completely prevent it. The slipping rate varies between 0.26% and 5.4%. Worldwide, up to 90% of these operations involve fixation of the fundus. In Germany, an increase in the slipping rate was observed after a decline in the application of fixation sutures.

The port tube is led through the 10 port access in the left upper abdomen in front of the abdominal wall. A skin incision is made to place the port. The fascia is then closed with sutures without damaging the tube. A subcutaneous pocket is then formed on the rectal sheath. The fascia is visualized with the dissecting scissors and partly blunt digital. A distance of 2–3 cm to the ribcage must be observed to avoid later mechanical irritation with considerable pain when bending. The port is fixed on the fascia with non-resorbable sutures. Some port implants are supplied with a fixation system. This allows the port to be easily fixed on the fascia with small hooks (■ Fig. 8.6). If the fixation is insufficient, there is a high risk of port torsion. The port tube must run loosely through the fascia into the abdominal cavity without kinking.

8.5 Aftercare, Band Filling

Filling of the band should only be done after healing, at the earliest 4–5 weeks postoperatively. Until then, the patient should remain on small amounts of liquid food, and food intake should be as slow as possible. After 4 weeks and completed wound healing, the port can usually be palpated subcutaneously and punctured with a Huber needle. Using a 10 ml syringe and physiological saline solution, the ligament is then successively filled under fluoroscopy until a thread-like tightness is evident. A sip of contrast medium should reach the stomach without any problems via 1–2 peristaltic waves. Finally, the correct implant position is checked and documented by fluoroscopy (■ Fig. 8.7).

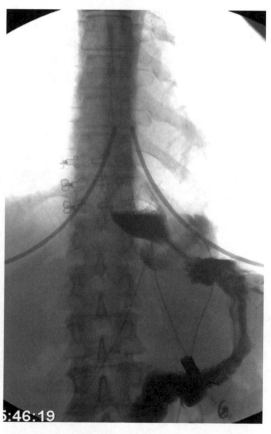

■ Fig. 8.7 Postoperative X-ray

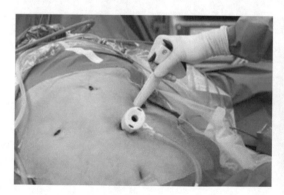

■ Fig. 8.6 Port placement

With appropriate experience, filling the belt is also possible without X-ray control. During slow filling, the patient must drink water until a sufficient feeling of tightness is achieved. It is crucial that after blocking, a sufficient fluid intake of 1.5–2 L per day is guaranteed. Often 2–3 appointments at intervals of 6–8 weeks are necessary to achieve a satisfactory banding for the patient. Thereafter, a check-up should be carried out at least once a year so that complications can be detected early on.

Early and late gastric band complications are described in detail in ▶ Sect. 14.7.

8.6 Pitfalls

- When preparing the retroesophageal tunnel, care must be taken to avoid dorsal esophageal injury.
- With a high-fat site, there is the danger of only charging the small-curvature fat pad with the goldfinger and thus misplacing the band. Therefore, the correct position-ing of the ligament should be checked by inserting a stomach tube before the ligament is closed.
- When applying the serosing sutures, there is a risk of damaging the implant with the back of the needle.
- An implantation that is too high, an esophageal banding, must be avoided in order to achieve a feeling of satiety by stretching the stomach wall during food intake.

Further Readings

Favretti F, Ashton D (2009) The gastric band: first-choice procedure for obesity surgery. World J Surg 33: 2039–2048

Singhal R, Bryant C (2010) Band slippage and erosion after laparoscopic gastric banding: a meta-analysis. Surg Endosc 24:2980–2986

Stroh C, Weiner R (2014) Revisional surgery and reopera-tions in obesity and metabolic surgery: data analysis of the German bariatric surgery registry 2005–2012. Chirurg 86:346–354

8

Sleeve Gastrectomy

J. Ordemann

Contents

© Springer-Verlag GmbH Germany, part of Springer Nature 2022
J. Ordemann, U. Elbelt (eds.), *Obesity and Metabolic Surgery*,
https://doi.org/10.1007/978-3-662-63227-7_9

Laparoscopic sleeve gastrectomy (LSG) became established in the 1990s. In the meantime, it has become one of the leading obesity surgeries and metabolic procedures in Germany and the USA.

The sleeve gastrectomy was originally used as part of biliopancreatic diversion with duodenal switch in extreme forms of obesity. Gagner et al. (2008) established the sleeve gastrectomy as a standalone operation and propagated it not only for weight reduction but also for metabolic surgery. The principle of action includes food restriction as well as hormonal mechanisms whose alteration leads to a faster feeling of satiety and a reduction in hunger (◘ Fig. 9.1).

Not only the excess weight of the patients is reduced, but also favourable results regarding type 2 diabetes, high blood pressure, sleep apnoea syndrome and other obesity-related diseases are achieved. In addition, patients report an improvement in their quality of life. Further advantages are the preservation

of the gastric passage. An oesophago-gastro-duodenoscopy can still be performed without problems.

A lack of vitamins/trace elements is rare, but supplementation is still recommended. In contrast to gastric banding and also gastric bypass surgery, sleeve gastrectomy is irreversible.

9.1 Trocar Placement

Generally, 5 trocars are needed. Their positioning should depend on the individual anatomy of the patient. The first trocar (T1; camera trocar, 12 mm) is placed approximately 15 cm below the xiphoid process 1–2 cm to the left of the median line (▶ Sect. 6.8). After the pneumoperitoneum has been created, the entire abdomen is inspected and injuries to intra-abdominal organs are excluded during trocar placement. The patient is then positioned in the anti-Trendelenburg position.

The second trocar (T2, 5 mm) is for the liver retractor and is inserted under visual control from the right lateral below the ribcage margin. The retractor is inserted and the left liver flap is lifted. The retractor is then fixed in place with a holding arm.

Now two further working trocars, T3 and T4 (12 mm each) are placed. These are placed to the left and right of the camera trocar in an imaginary crescent-shaped line to the xyphoid. The left working trocar (T3), as seen from the surgeon, is to be positioned in such a way that the linear cutter needed later does not approach the antrum too steeply. Thus, trocar T3 must be placed somewhat lower and more laterally in the right epigastrium.

Finally, another 5 mm trocar (T5) is inserted into the left lateral upper abdomen (◘ Fig. 9.2).

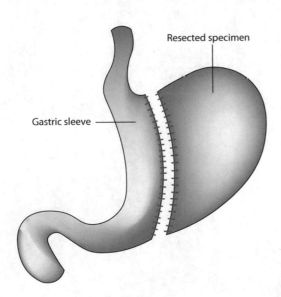

Resected specimen

Gastric sleeve

◘ **Fig. 9.1**   Sleeve gastrectomy

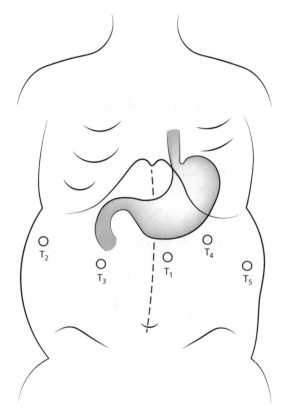

Fig. 9.2　Trocar placement

9.2　Exploration

Exploration and presentation of the surgical site are an important part of the operation. All quadrants of the abdomen must be inspected. Adhesions, inflammations, ascites, tumors, liver and spleen size are important additional findings that can change the surgical plan or even make it necessary to terminate the operation. When inspecting the hiatus region, special attention should be paid to the presence of a possible hiatal hernia. If such a hernia is present, the stomach must be reduced and the hiatus narrowed.

9.3　Dissection

Before starting the dissection, a calibration tube should be placed by the anesthesiologist. Our centre uses a 36 Fr. tube for this purpose. The stomach should be completely emptied at

the beginning of the dissection. It is then lifted with an atraumatic grasping forceps (T3) in the area of the corpus. The lig. gastrocolicum is grasped via T5 and carefully tightened. The ultrasound dissector is introduced through T4, the gastrocolic ligament is severed close to the stomach (■ Fig. 9.3) and thus the bursa omentalis (■ Fig. 9.4) is opened.

Then the greater curvature of the stomach is carefully dissected in the direction of the fundus. The fundus (■ Fig. 9.5) is mobilized and the short gastric vessels are divided using ultrasound dissector.

> ❗ Too much traction on the fundus can lead to rupture of the short gastric vessels or even injury to the spleen. Therefore, special caution is required.

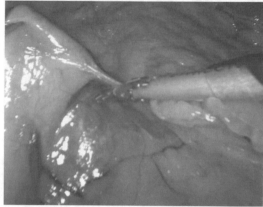

Fig. 9.3　Settling of the gastrocolic ligament near the stomach

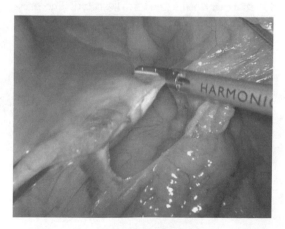

Fig. 9.4　Opened bursa omentalis

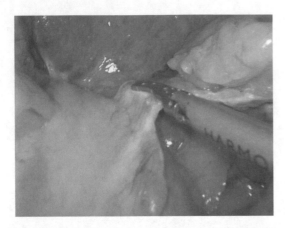

Fig. 9.5 Funduscap with spleen

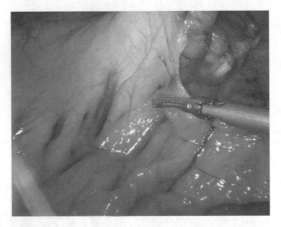

Fig. 9.6 Dissection of the gastrocolic ligament to distal

The fundus cap is prepared up to the hiatus. By careful mobilization the complete presentation of the left diaphragm is performed. Dorsal adhesions must be dissected. The presence of a hiatal hernia must be excluded.

The pylorus is then displayed. In order not to obstruct gastric emptying after sleeve gastrectomy, the preparation should not reach directly to the pylorus. A distance of 3–6 cm is recommended. For further preparation, the middle corpus area and the gastrocolic ligament are lifted with atraumatic grasping forceps and dissected distally (**Fig. 9.6**). The posterior wall of the stomach is carefully exposed and any adhesions between stomach and pancreas are dissected.

! It is essential to ensure that neither the duodenum nor the rear wall of the stomach or the capsule of the pancreas are damaged by thermal injuries.

9.4 Gastric Tube Calibration

If the calibration tube has not already been placed as described above (▸ Sect. 9.3), it should be inserted orally via the oesophagus into the stomach at this point at the latest (**Fig. 9.7**).

> **Practical Tip**
>
> The surgeon should make sure that no additional stomach tube has been placed unnoticed by the anaesthetist.

The calibration tube must run parallel to the lesser curve, the end of the calibration tube should be in front of the pylorus.

> **Practical Tip**
>
> If the calibration tube has holes, the anaesthetist must disconnect the tube to ensure that the tube can be easily moved.

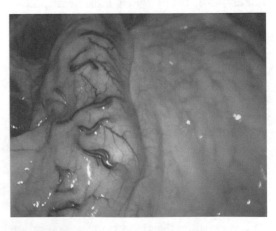

Fig. 9.7 Advancing the calibration tube

9.5 **Resection**

The linear cutter (green cartridge) is placed through T3 trocar approximately 3–6 cm from the pylorus. The linear cutter should be placed carefully with slight pulling of the stomach laterally (■ Fig. 9.8). If the linear cutter is closed, the stomach tube must not be grasped. The anaesthetist is requested to carefully push the gastric tube back and forth. The closed linear cutter should not be released immediately. It is recommended to wait 15 s to reduce tissue edema by compression. The linear cutter is then released, then opened and carefully removed.

Now the resection is continued parallel to the calibration tube (■ Fig. 9.9). It is recommended to use a total of two green cartridges

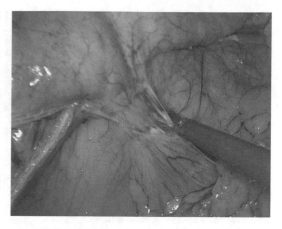

■ Fig. 9.10 Dissecting adhesions

(2 mm). Afterwards blue cartridges (1.5 mm) are used, as the stomach wall becomes thinner toward the upper part of the stomach. After each closure of the linear cutter the anaesthetist should be asked to carefully move the stomach tube back and forth. This prevents the sleeve from becoming too narrow.

The posterior wall of the stomach should be checked regularly. Dorsal adhesions (■ Fig. 9.10) must be dissected. They can be cut through with scissors without risk of bleeding. Attention must be paid to injuries to larger vessels and the pancreatic capsule.

Twisting of the stomach and cross-stapling must be avoided at all costs. For easy access to the proximal fundus, the linear cutter can also be inserted via T1 or T4. Care must be taken to ensure that the entire fundus is resected.

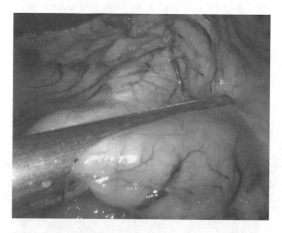

■ Fig. 9.8 Attached linear cutter

Practical Tip
A gastric sleeve that is too narrow with a "relatively" wide residual fundus can lead to increased stress on the fresh staple suture line due to the funnel effect.

It is not necessary to overstitch the whole staple line. However, some authors recommend overstitching in both the antrum and the angle of His to reduce the rate of leakage. If necessary, the staple suture can be reinforced with individual clips, and minor bleeding can be stopped in this way (■ Fig. 9.11).

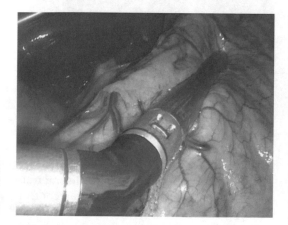

■ Fig. 9.9 Formation of the sleeve

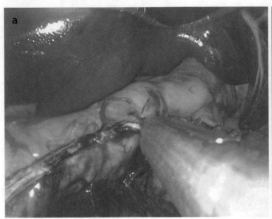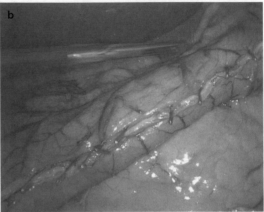

◧ **Fig. 9.11   a** Clipping of minor bleeding. **b** Staple line supplied with clips

9.6 Test for Staple Line Insufficiency

Finally, the anaesthetist is asked to retract the calibration tube by 2–3 cm. The stomach is closed with an atraumatic clamp proximal to the pylorus. The gastric sleeve is then filled quickly with approximately 100 ml methylene blue solution through the calibration tube until the gastric sleeve is stretched. Particular attention must be paid to leaks, especially at the distal and proximal end of the gastric sleeve. The calibration tube is then removed under visual control.

9.7 Removal of the Resected Specimen

The sleeve gastrectomy specimen is removed via an extended trocar incision in the area of T4. The skin incision is extended by 1 cm and the external fascia is then exposed. This is also incised by about 1 cm. Then the trocar is removed and the incision is dilated with the help of two fingers. Now, under camera control and with a grasping forceps, the resected specimen is grasped at its distal end and carefully extracted over the trocar incision. Finally, the specimen can be safely removed by moving it slightly back and forth. Care must be taken that the pull on the specimen is not too strong to avoid perforation of the gas-

tric specimen. The use of a recovery bag is not necessary. The infection rate in the recovery area is not increased by this procedure. The extended fascial incision must be closed with a suture.

9.8 Finishing the Operation

After closure of the incision, a final check of the surgical site is necessary. In particular, bleeding from the staple suture line and the abdominal wall must be excluded.

> **Practical Tip**
>
> If necessary, the anaesthetist can be asked to slightly raise the blood pressure with medication to make any bleeding detectable.

Particular attention should be paid to bleeding in the area of the spleen, the staple sutures and the back wall of the stomach.

The insertion of a drainage tube is usually not necessary. However, if a drainage tube is inserted, it is recommended to place it above T5.

At the end of the operation the liver retractor must be removed under visual control. The trocars are also removed under visual control. The incisions are checked for bleeding. Closure of the fascia in the area of the trocar incisions is usually not necessary. The skin is stapled or treated with intracutaneous skin sutures.

9.9 Pitfalls

- A hiatal hernia must be ruled out; if such a hernia is present, the hiatus must be constricted with a hiatoplasty.
- The left diaphragm should be completely exposed.
- Only one calibration tube may be inserted. It must be ensured that the anaesthetist has not placed a second stomach tube intragastrally.
- During the preparation, the tension on the fundus must not be too much to avoid injury to the vessels and the spleen.
- Dorsal adhesions must be dissected in order to avoid twisting of the sleeve gastrectomy.
- A check of the staple line for bleeding and hematomas is necessary; a staple line that is not completely closed leads to staple suture failure.

References

Gagner M, Gumbs AA, Milone L et al (2008) Laparoscopic sleeve gastrectomy for the super-super-obese. Surg Today 38:399–403

Further Readings

Agarwal S, Kini SU, Herron DM (2007) Laparoscopic sleeve gastrectomy for morbid obesity: a review. Surg Obes Relat Dis 3:189–194

ASMBS Online Statements/Guidelines (2012) Updated position statement on sleeve gastrectomy as a bariatric procedure. Surg Obes Relat Dis 3:573–576

Brethauer SA, Hammel J, Schauer PR (2009) Systematic review of sleeve gastrectomy as a staging and primary bariatric operation. Surg Obes Relat Dis 5:469–475

Buchwald H, Avidor Y, Braunwald E et al (2004) Bariatric surgery. A systematic review and meta analysis. JAMA 292:1774–1737

Daskalakis M, Berdan Y, Theodoridous S, Weigand G, Weiner RA (2011) Impact of surgeon experience and buttress material on postoperative complications after laparoscopic sleeve gastrectomy. Surg Endosc 25:88–97

Gagner M, Deitel M, Kalberer TL et al (2009) The second international consensus summit for sleeve gastrectomy. Surg Obes Relat Dis 5:476–485

Himpens J, Dobbeleir J, Peeters G (2010) Long-term results of laparoscopic sleeve gastrectomy for obesity. Ann Surg 252:319–324

Khan S, Rock K, Bhaskara A, Qu W et al (2016) Trends in bariatric surgery from 2008 to 2012. Am J Surg 211:1041–1046

Rosenthal RJ (2012) International Sleeve Gastrectomy Expert Panel Consensus Statement: best practice guidelines based on experience of >12,000 cases. Surg Obes Relat Dis 8:8–19

Rubin M, Yehoshua RT, Stein M et al (2008) Laparoscopic sleeve gastrectomy with minimal morbidity: early results in 120 morbidly obese patients. Obes Surg 18:1567–1570

Runke N, Colombo-Benkmann M, Hüttl TP et al (2011) Evidence-based German guidelines for surgery for obesity. Int J Colorectal Dis 26:397–404

Schauer PE, Kashyap SR, Wolski K, Brethauer SA et al (2012) Bariatric surgery versus intensive medical therapy in obese patients with diabetes. NEJM 366:1567–1576

Weiner RA, Weiner S, Pomhoff I et al (2007) Laparoscopic sleeve gastrectomy—influence of sleeve size and resected gastric volume. Obes Surg 17:1297–1305

Laparoscopic, Proximal Roux-en-Y Gastric Bypass

J. Ordemann

Contents

© Springer-Verlag GmbH Germany, part of Springer Nature 2022
J. Ordemann, U. Elbelt (eds.), *Obesity and Metabolic Surgery*,
https://doi.org/10.1007/978-3-662-63227-7_10

10.1 Trocar Placement

For the application of laparoscopic gastric bypass five trocars are generally sufficient. However, a sixth or seventh trocar can be placed in particularly demanding surgical conditions.

The positioning of the trocars should be modified according to the individual anatomy of the patient. In general, the first trocar (T1; camera trocar, 12 mm) is placed approximately 15 cm below the xypoid, 1–2 cm to the left of the median line. (▶ Sect. 6.8). After the pneumoperitoneum has been created, the entire abdominal cavity is inspected and injuries to intra-abdominal organs are excluded during trocar placement. The patient is then positioned in a reserve Trendelenburg position.

The second trocar (T2, 5 mm) is for the liver retractor and is inserted under visual control from the right lateral below the ribcage margin. The retractor is inserted and the

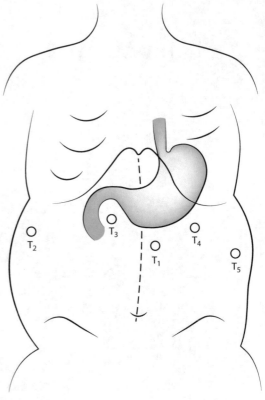

Fig. 10.2 Trocar placement

left liver flap is lifted. The retractor is then fixed in place with a holding arm.

Next, two further working trocars T3 and T4 (12 mm each) are placed. These are placed to the left and right of the camera trocar in an imaginary crescent-shaped line to the xyphoid. Finally, a further 5 mm trocar (T5) is inserted into the left lateral upper abdomen (▣ Fig. 10.2).

10.2 Exploration

The exploration of the entire abdominal cavity is an important part of the operation. Adhesions, inflammations, ascites, tumors, liver and spleen size are important additional findings that can change the surgical plan or even make it necessary to terminate the operation. The gallbladder and the hiatus region should especially be carefully checked.

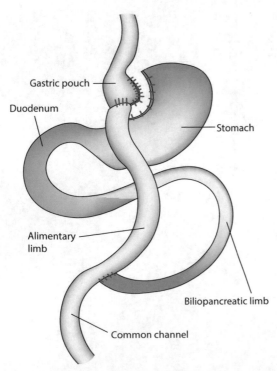

Gastric pouch
Duodenum
Stomach
Alimentary limb
Biliopancreatic limb
Common channel

Fig. 10.1 Proximal gastric bypass

10

In cases of pronounced abdominal obesity, it is important to check whether the future alimentary limb can be lifted to the future pouch without tension. If this is not possible—even after dividing the omentum—it is recommended that a sleeve gastrectomy be performed (the patient must be informed about this preoperatively).

10.3 Creating the Gastric Pouch

First the angle of His is displayed (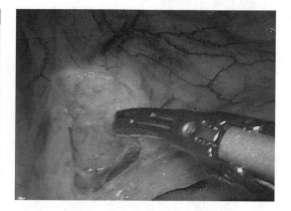 Fig. 10.3). Then the peritoneal coating is opened with the ultrasound scissors. The left crus of diaphragm is partially displayed. If there is a hiatal hernia with or without herniation of the gastric fundus, it is essential that the fundus be repositioned and the hiatal hernia is treated with anterior hiatoplasty.

The stomach is then grasped over the trocar T5 with atraumatic grasping forceps and lifted by the assistant. Now the dissection of the hepatogastric ligament (lesser omentum) between the second and third vessel below the gastroesophageal junction takes place as close to the stomach wall as possible (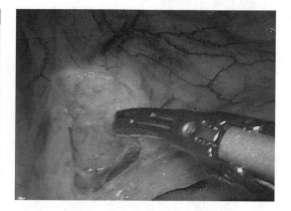 Fig. 10.4). The dissection should be performed very subtly to avoid injury to the left gastric artery or its lateral branches. The bursa omentalis must definitely be opened.

Fig. 10.4 Dissection close to the stomach

Even minor bleeding should be avoided at all costs, as bleeding into the lesser omentum makes safe preparation considerably more difficult.

Adhesions are found more frequently in the area of the posterior stomach wall. These must be sealed and cut through. The preparation of the posterior stomach wall must be done extremely carefully to avoid injuries in the area of the pancreas and the spleen.

At this time at the latest, a tube (36 French) should be placed orally into the stomach for calibration.

Care must be taken not to insert two tubes into the stomach (an oral calibration tube and a nasal tube). The calibration tube must not form loops.

Once the bursa omentalis (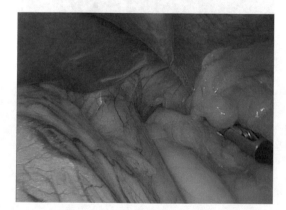 Fig. 10.5) is opened, the stomach is partially cut through horizontally with a linear cutter from the small curvature. The linear cutter should be inserted through the left 12 mm trocar (T3) (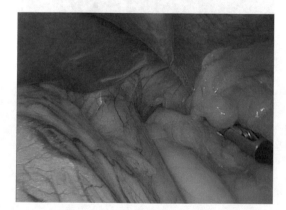 Fig. 10.6). Care should be taken that the linear cutter is not too steeply directed towards

Fig. 10.3 Angle of His

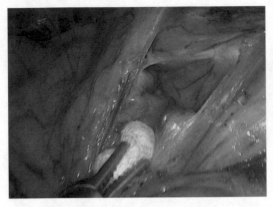

Fig. 10.5 Bursa omentalis

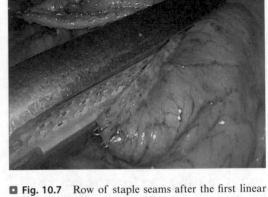

Fig. 10.7 Row of staple seams after the first linear cutter is triggered

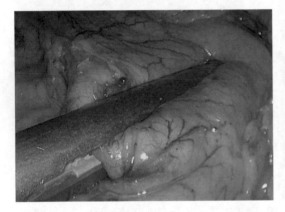

Fig. 10.6 Placement of the first linear cutter

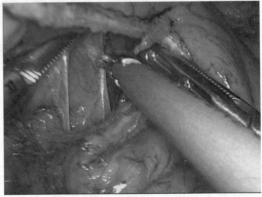

Fig. 10.8 Dissecting dorsal adhesions from the stomach pouch

10

the stomach and can be inserted without resistance. If a 60 mm linear cutter is used, do not use the entire length of the cartridge, but only a length of 30–45 mm. It is recommended to use a blue cartridge (1.5 mm). The calibration tube must be retracted before the stapling begins and must not be within the range of the staple line.

After triggering the stapling device, the staple line (■ Fig. 10.7) must be checked for bleeding. Afterwards the dorsal side of the pouch is released from adhesions (■ Fig. 10.8).

The second linear cutter is now placed at right angles to the primary resection plane in the direction up to the angle of His (■ Fig. 10.9). In general, 2–3 cartridges are sufficient to completely cut through the fundus.

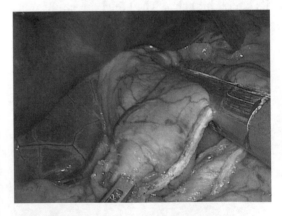

Fig. 10.9 Attaching the second linear cutter

It is absolutely necessary to cut through the stomach completely in order to avoid gastric-gastric fistula.

10.4 Measurement of the Intestine

10.4.1 Dividing the Greater Omentum

Dividing the greater omentum is not always necessary. However, in cases of severe abdominal obesity, it has proven to be advantageous in order to enable a tension-free gastrojejunostomy.

Then the greater omentum is lifted into the upper abdomen and divide in cranial direction using the ultrasound dissector. Divide the omentum up to the transverse colon. Bleeding must be meticulously avoided as it is often difficult to detect during the course of the operation.

10.4.2 Mobilizing the First Jejunum Loop

The meso of the colon is then grasped transversely and carefully lifted. The ligament of Treitz (◘ Fig. 10.10) must be clearly identified. The first jejunal loop is grasped with atraumatic grasping forceps and a distance of approximately 50 cm is measured. The

measured jejunal loop is moved to the left (patient's left side). It is then moved antecolic-antegastric to the upper abdomen and should be brought up to the pouch without tension. The oral loop (patient's left side) is the future biliopancreatic limb, the aboral loop (patient's right side) is the future alimentary limb. It's obligatory to avoid a mix-up of the two loops.

10.5 Gastrojejunal Anastomosis

Gastrojejunostomy can be performed using various techniques. In addition to linear stapled anastomosis, there is the possibility of circular stapled anastomosis and completely hand-sewn anastomosis. Our centre prefers the linear stapled anastomosis, as it can be performed quickly and results in few complications.

10.5.1 Linear Stapled Anastomosis

The ultrasound dissector is used to open the stomach pouch on the posterior side (◘ Fig. 10.11). The stomach wall must be completely opened.

The raised intestine is carefully opened on its lateral front side with the ultrasonic scissors. The back of the small intestine loop should then be checked directly for thermal damage.

The linear stapled anastomosis is applied through trocar 3, the branches of the stapler

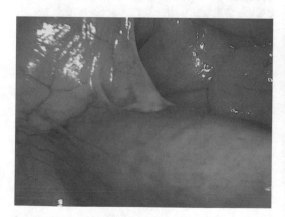

◘ **Fig. 10.10** Ligament of Treitz

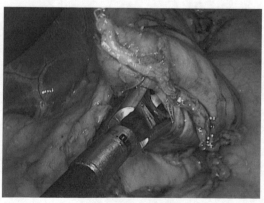

◘ **Fig. 10.11** Opened stomach pouch

are first inserted into the small intestine and then as atraumatically as possible into the pouch (◻ Fig. 10.12). The decisive factor is that the future biliopancreatic limb is on the patient's left side and the future alimentary limb is on the patient's right side. Then it should again be ensured that there is no mix-up between the two limbs.

The linear stapled anastomosis must not be applied too far into the pouch and should not exceed 30 mm. A blue cartridge is generally used for the anastomosis. After removal of the stapler, the stapled line is checked for bleeding both extra- and intraluminally. Intra- and also extra-luminal bleeding in the area of the stapled line can usually be safely treated with clips.

The enterotomy is closed with a single-layer running suture (3-0 thread) (◻ Fig. 10.13). All wall layers should be completely covered.

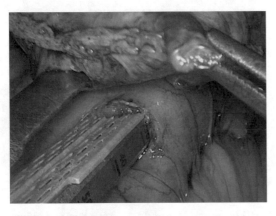

◻ **Fig. 10.12** Inserted stapler cartridge into the intestine and pouch

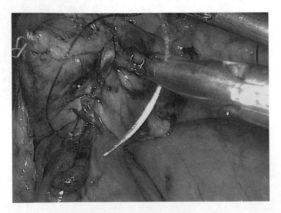

◻ **Fig. 10.13** Closing the gastroenterostoma

The anastomosis is splinted with a calibration tube in order to avoid suturing the anastomosis too tightly. It is recommended to reinforce the single layer running suture with a second or with single button sutures.

10.5.2 Circular Stapled Anastomosis

Circular stapled anastomosis can be applied using different techniques. The main difference is the introduction of the pressure plate required for circular stapled anastomosis into the stomach pouch: it can be performed either orally or intraabdominally.

Pressure Plate Inserted from the Abdomen

The left staple corner of the pouch is opened with the ultrasonic scissors. The pouch opening is then dilated with atraumatic grasping forceps. Then a circular, all-layer tobacco pouch suture is applied.

The circular stapler (25 mm) is guided from the left laterally (in the area of the T5 trocar, which has to be removed for a short time) through the dilated trocar incision to the abdominal cavity. The dilated incision should be closed with clamps to avoid CO_2 leakage. The pressure plate of the stapler is extended and released from the stapler. The stapler is then removed and the trocar is reinserted into the incision site.

The pressure plate is carefully inserted into the stomach pouch. This requires patience and practice. The pressure plate inserted into the pouch is fixed with the tobacco pouch seam. This is tightened and knotted. If the closure is not complete, an additional circular seam must be applied.

Now the renewed search for the jejunum limb from the ligament of Treitz is carried out as described above. The intestine loop should be led tension-free up to the pouch. The loop coming from the patient's left side is the future biliopancreatic limb, the loop leading to the right is the future alimentary limb. The intestine is opened with the ultrasound scissors. The circular stapler is then reintroduced through the incision site of T5 (trocar must be removed briefly as described above). Then the entire stapler head is placed in the intestine lumen. Injury to the intestinal wall must be avoided. Once the stapler head is safely placed in the small intestine, the tip of the stapler can be extended and the small intestine perforated. The intestine should under no circumstances be unintentionally perforated more than once. Then the advanced mandrel of the circular stapler is connected to the plate. The system is retracted and the circular stapler anastomosis is applied. After careful removal of the circular stapler, it is recommended to check that the intestine wall ring and the gastric wall ring are complete. These must be intact.

Pressure Plate Inserted Orally

The pressure plate required for circular stapled suture anastomosis is fixed to a stomach tube. The stomach tube is then carefully passed through the mouth into the oesophagus and finally into the stomach pouch. Then a small incision is made in the pouch using the ultrasonic scissors and the stomach tube is guided out of the pouch. The gastric tube is pulled completely intraabdominally and thus the tip of the pressure plate is pulled through the small incision. As soon as the pressure plate is placed in the correct position, the stomach tube is released from the tip of the pressure plate and completely removed through the trocar.

Then the circular stapler anastomosis, which is as free of tension as possible, is performed as described above.

10.5.3 Hand Sewn Anastomosis

The jejunum limb—as shown in detail above— is first fixed to the stomach pouch with corner seams parallel to the horizontal row of staple seams. Then the first continuous suture of the posterior wall is applied with an absorbable 3-0 thread. The pouch and the jejunum loop are then opened to a length of 1.5–2 cm either with an electric hook or with the ultrasonic scissors. Then a running suture is performed through all the layers of the posterior wall with an absorbable 3-0 thread. A calibration tube is then inserted into the intestine through

the stomach pouch. Without grasping the calibration tube, the anterior wall is closed with a running suture. It is recommended to reinforced the first running suture with a second.

10.6 Measuring the Alimentary Loop

After gastrojejunostomy, the alimentary limb is measured. This is done with marked, atraumatic grasping forceps or by inserting a measuring tape. The length of the limb should be between 120 and 150 cm for proximal gastric bypass. It is important that the alimentary limb is guided to the patient's ride side.

10.7 Jejunojejunostomy

The jejunojejunostomy is usually performed as a wide side-to-side stapler anastomosis. The loops to be anastomised are opened antimesenterally with the ultrasound dissector. The enterotomy (◘ Fig. 10.14) in the area of the biliopancreatic loop should be performed approximately 4–6 cm below the gastrojejunostomy.

A linear cutter with a white 60 mm cartridge is used to apply the anastomosis. The linear cutter is guided through the T3 trocar into the abdominal cavity and the branches are carefully inserted into both parallel limbs. After application of the anastomosis, the sta-

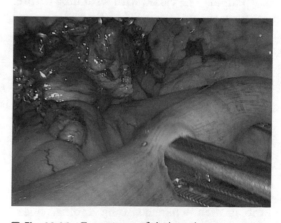

◘ **Fig. 10.14** Enterotomy of the intestine

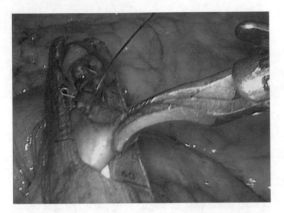

◻ Fig. 10.15   Closure of the enterotomy using a stapler

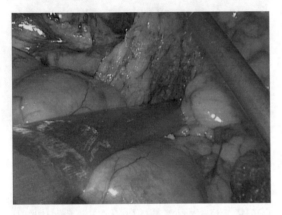

◻ Fig. 10.16   Dividing the biliopancreatic loop

pled sutures are checked intraluminally and extraluminally for bleeding.

The enterotomy is now brought together by an adapting single-button suture and closed with one or two additional white cartridges (◻ Fig. 10.15). However, the enterotomy can also be closed with a running suture.

10.8 Dividing of the Biliopancreatic Loop

After completion of the jejunojejunostomie, the biliopancreatic loop must now be divided under the stomach pouch (◻ Fig. 10.16). In order to do this, the meso of the biliopancreatic loop must be carefully opened about 3 cm from the gastrojejunostomy. Thermal damage of the small intestine must be avoided. The limb is then separated using another linear cutter (white cartridge).

10.9 Testing the Gastro-entero Anastomosis for Leaks

In order to test for leaks of the gastrojejunostomy, the alimentary loop below the anastomosis is closed with an atraumatic clamp. The anaesthetist is requested to apply methylene blue solution into the stomach pouch until the anastomosis is stretched. The entire row of sutures (including the posterior wall) should be checked for leaks.

10.10 Closing the Mesentery

Since internal herniations may occur, it is recommended that artificial openings in the mesentery (Peterson space) be closed with non-absorbable sutures.

10.11 Finishing the Operation

At the end of the operation, the entire surgical area should be checked for bleeding and possible injuries. A drainage tube is usually not necessary. However, it is recommended for high-risk patients or patients with an increased tendency of bleeding. The inserted liver retractor is removed under visual control. The trocars are then also removed under visual control. Closure of the fascia of the trocar incisions is usually not necessary. If a circular stapler was used for gastrojejunostomy, the fascia of the incision must be securely closed. The skin is then stapled or treated with sutures.

10.12 Pitfalls

- A hiatal hernia must be ruled out; if such a hernia is present, the hiatus must be constricted.
- The preparation of the pouch must be done close to the stomach to protect the vessels supplying the pouch.
- Bleeding in the area of the stomach wall should be stopped immediately to avoid haematomas which could complicate the preparation.

10

- A complete transection of the stomach during formation of the pouch is necessary to avoid gastro-gastric fistula postoperatively.
- The ligament of Treitz must be clearly displayed in order to avoid a mix-up of the limbs.
- A secure hemostasis when cutting the omentum is crucial because massive bleeding can occur here.
- Undetected defects and perforations of the small intestine must be avoided.
- The application of a wide jejunojejunostomy is necessary to avoid a stenosis.

Further Readings

Dillemans B, Sakran N, Van Cauwenberge S et al (2009a) Standardization of the fully stapled laparoscopic Roux-en13Y gastric bypass for obesity reduces early immediate postoperative morbidity and mortality: a single center study on 2606 patients. Obes Surg 19:1355–1364

Dillemans B, Sakran N, Van Cauwenberge S et al (2009b) Standardization of the fully stapled laparoscopic Roux-en-Y gastric bypass for obesity reduces early immediate postoperative morbidity and mortality: a single center study on 2606 patients. Obes Surg 19:1355–1364

Higa K, Boone K, Arteaga Gonzales I et al (2007) Mesenteric closure in laparoscopic gastric bypass: surgical technique and literature review. Cir Esp 2:77–88

Lee S, Davies A, Bahal S et al (2014) Comparison of gastrojejunal anastomosis techniques in laparoscopic Roux-en-Y gastric bypass: gastrojejunal stricture rate and effect on subsequent weight loss. Obes Surg 24:1425–1429

Madan AK, Harper JL, Tichansky DS (2008) Techniques of laparoscopic gastric bypass: on-line survey of American Society for Bariatric Surgery practicing surgeons. Surg Obes Relat Dis 4:166–172

Mason EE, Ito C (1967) Gastric bypass in obesity. Surg Clin North Am 47:1345–1351

Schauer PR, Ikramuddin S, Hamad G et al (2003b) Laparoscopic gastric bypass surgery: current technique. J Laparoendosc Adv Surg Tech 13:229–239

Schauer PR, Ikramuddin S, Hamad G, Gourash W (2003a) The learning curve for laparoscopic Roux-en-Y gastric bypass is 100 cases. Surg Endosc 17:212–215

Szomstein S, Whipple OC, Zundel N, Cal P, Rosenthal R (2006) Laparoscopic Roux-en-Y gastric bypass with linear cutter technique: comparison of four-row versus six-row cartridge in creation anastomosis. Surg Obes Relat Dis 2:431–434

Weiner RA (2008) Obesity principles of surgical therapy. Chirurg 79:826–828

Weiner RA, Blnco-Engert R, Winterberg U (2003) Laparoskopischer Roux-en-Y-Magenbypass–Technik und Komplikationen. Chir Gastroenterol 19:62–69

Wittgrove AC, Clark GW, Tremblay LJ (1994) Laparoscopic gastric bypass, Roux-en-Y: preliminary report of five cases. Obes Surg 4:4353–4357

Omega-Loop Bypass (One-Anastomosis Bypass, Mini-Gastric Bypass)

T. P. Hüttl, P. Stauch, and O. Dietl

Contents

© Springer-Verlag GmbH Germany, part of Springer Nature 2022
J. Ordemann, U. Elbelt (eds.), *Obesity and Metabolic Surgery*,
https://doi.org/10.1007/978-3-662-63227-7_11

The one-anastomosis bypass was developed by Rutledge in 1997. A report of a large case series that included more than 1200 patients was published in 2001 (Rutledge 2001). In recent years, this technique has become established as one procedure within the spectrum of bariatric surgery (◘ Table 11.1, ► Sect. 11.10). In the current surgical S3 guideline (Runkel et al. 2011) it is described as an effective procedure, but is not yet listed as a standard procedure like gastric banding, sleeve gastrectomy, Roux-en-Y gastric bypass and BPD-DS (◘ Fig. 11.1).

The term (laparoscopic) "mini-gastric bypass" (MGB/LMGB) seems to be confusing (Carbajo and Luque-de-León 2015). In fact, it is a "real" gastric bypass, not a "partial" or an "incomplete" bypass. The procedure is also known as "one-anastomosis gastric bypass" (OAGB) or "single-anastomosis gastric bypass" (SAGB). In the following text we use the original term from Rutledge: "MGB" or "omega-loop gastric bypass".

◘ Table 11.1   Current results of the omega-loop bypass

Author	N	Start	Major complica-tions (%)	Mor-tality (%)	Initial BMI (kg/m^2)	BMI (kg/m^2) at follow-up	% EWL	% Remission D. M. type 2
Rutledge et al. (2005)	2410	1997	5.9	0.08	46.0	–	–	–
Lee et al. (2012)	1163	2001	1.8	0.17	41.4	27.7	72.9	93.0
Carbajo et al. (2005)	209	2002	0.9	48.0	–	–	75.0	–
Peraglie (2008)	16	2005	0	0	62.4	–	65.0	–
Noun et al. (2012)	1000	2005	3.4	0	42.5	28.4	68.6	–
Chakhtoura et al. (2008)	100	2006	7.0	0	46.9	31.9	63.0	–
Darabi et al. (2013)	20	2010	0	0	49.5	33.4	66.9	50.0
Musella et al. (2013)	974	2006	2.0	0.2	48.0	28.0	77.0	86.0
Kular et al. (2014)	1054	2007	1.3	0.18	43.2	25.9	87.0	93.0
Clarke et al. (2013)	156	2005	2.6	0	46.0	26.0	89.0	–
Total or average	**7102**		**3.4**	**0.14**	**44.7**	**27.6**	**74.9**	**90.6**

Mod. according to Lee and Lin (2014)

BMI body mass index, *DM* diabetes mellitus, *EWL* excess weight loss

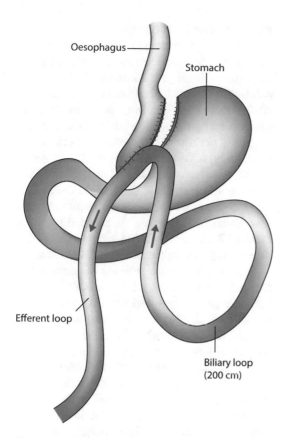

Oesophagus

Stomach

Efferent loop

Biliary loop
(200 cm)

◨ **Fig. 11.1**   Omega-loop gastric bypass

11.1 **Indication**

⊕ A distinction has to be made between the omega-loop bypass as a primary operation ("stand-alone procedure") or a conversion operation ("redo-operation").

▪ **Primary Operation**

Rutledge developed the omega-loop bypass aiming at developing an effective and low-risk procedure which is less complicated and faster to perform than a traditional gastric bypass. The laparoscopic formation of the gastrojejunostomy is easier to perform with the omega-loop bypass because there is less tension on the anastomosis. In addition, the gastrojejunostomy is accessible by endoscopy. The malabsorptive effect of an omega-loop bypass is more pronounced compared to a Roux-en-Y gastric bypass.

▪ **Secondary Operation**

In Europe, the omega-loop bypass is increasingly replacing BPD-DS and Roux-en-Y gastric bypass as a secondary surgical procedure. Experts estimate an omega-loop bypass to be advantageous compared to a Roux-en-Y gastric bypass in terms of a more favorable effect on type 2 diabetes mellitus with a reduced risk of developing a dumping syndrome. In addition, the surgical procedure is easier to perform than BPD-DS surgery. Furthermore, a bile acid malabsorption occurs if at all rarely. Further studies are needed to learn whether conversion of a sleeve gastrectomy (high-pressure procedure) to an omega-loop bypass (low-pressure procedure) leads to sufficient improvement of symptomatic gastroesophageal reflux. Currently, conversion of sleeve gastrectomy to gastric bypass is still the standard redo surgical procedure for the treatment of symptomatic reflux disease (◨ Fig. 11.2).

Since no additional small bowel anastomosis is necessary for this type of operation, anastomotic bleeding is less frequent and the unlikely case of bleeding the gastrojejunostomy is accessible by endoscopy.

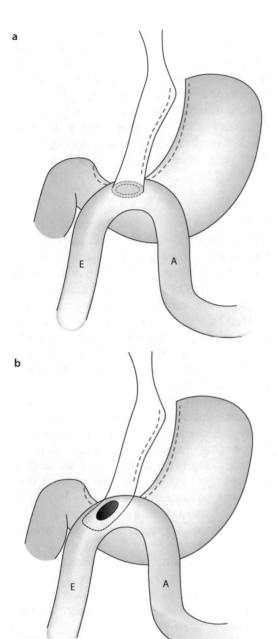

Fig. 11.2 a, b Mini-gastric bypass. Schematic representation of an omega-loop gastric bypass. The biliary limb measures 200 cm from Treitz ligament. **a** End-to-side reconstruction (original technique). **b** Side-to-side reconstruction: the afferent loop is higher than the efferent loop, if necessary by means of additional Kappeller sutures (*E* efferent loop, *A* afferent loop). (From Lee and Lin 2014)

11.2 Trocar Placement

The operation is performed with the patient in a supine position, also known as the French position. The patient is set in an approximately 20–30° anti-Trendelenburg position with the surgeon standing between the patient's legs.

For creation of a pneumoperitoneum (18 mmHg) a Verres needle is used. The Verres needle is inserted directly below the left costal arch slightly medial of the midclavicular line. After creation of the pneumoperitoneum the first trocar (optic trocar) is inserted approximately 17–20 cm below the xiphoid on the left side through the rectus abdominis muscle.

The first look after entering the abdomen is focused on the correct placement of the Verres needle, which is removed from the situs under visual control, also the pneumoperitoneum is reduced to 12–14 mmHg. Under visual control additional trocars are placed as follows: a 5 or 12 mm trocar on the right side for later insertion of a liver retractor or paddle—depending on the liver size. In the case of a small left liver lobe, the insertion of this trocar is not always necessary. Subsequently, two 5 mm trocars are placed in the left upper abdomen for the right hand of the surgeon and for the assistant. In addition, a 12 mm trocar is placed lateral or through the rectus abdominis muscle in the right upper abdomen for the use of a 12 mm stapler-cutter.

With a diagnostic all-round view, relevant adhesions and absolute or relative contraindications such as liver cirrhosis are excluded. Pylorus and angular incisure are identified, the hiatus is inspected for the presence of a diaphragmatic hernia, and the procedure is terminated, changed (sleeve gastrectomy), or modified (e.g., additional hiatoplasty) if necessary.

11.3 Dissection

At the angle of His, the gastrophrenic membranes are cut through with hooks and/or dissector (analogous to gastric banding, Roux-en-Y gastric bypass), this later facilitates the correct placement of the linear stapler when the gastric sleeve is created.

According to the original technique, the omentum minus is fenestrated just above the angular incisure at the boundary between the gastric antrum and corpus. The fenestration is performed with ultrasonic scissors. This is the latest possible time point for the anaesthetist to place a 12 mm calibration tube in the stomach.

11.4 Pouch

With careful observance of the calibration tube, the stomach is partially cut horizontally with the stapler-cutter using a green or gold cartridge. Then, similar to a sleeve gastrectomy, the tubular pouch is formed parallel to the small curve up to the angle of His. Occasionally, adhesions have to be carefully removed under visual control. The Vv. gastricae breves are preserved.

11.5 Measuring the Bypass Length

The small intestine is measured with a measuring tape or with markings on the grasping forceps and marked at 200 cm from the Treitz ligament. This results in a significantly more pronounced malabsorption compared to Roux-en-Y gastric bypass with a 50 cm biliary loop. In the case of super obese patients (BMI > 50 kg/m^2), some authors favour a loop length of up to 300 cm. In contrast, in lower-grade obese patients undergoing metabolic surgery, loop lengths of 150 cm are described (reviewed by Lee and Lin 2014).

11.6 Anastomosis

The anastomosis is performed antecolically as an end-to-side hand-sewn anastomosis or as a side-to-side anastomosis (functional end-to-side anastomosis) using a linear stapler (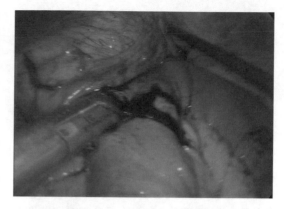 Fig. 11.3).

After suturing the posterior wall, the anterior wall of the hand-sewn anastomosis should not be sutured until the calibration tube has been pushed forward to avoid stenosis (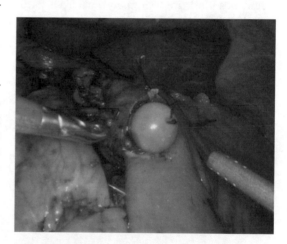 Fig. 11.4). In case of stapler anastomosis, bleeding of the staple suture has to be excluded before closing of the incisions.

Again, the incision can be closed by means of a linear stapler or by hand-sewn suture (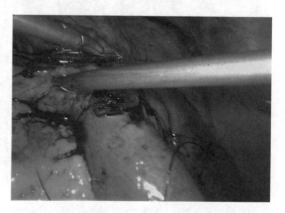 Fig. 11.5). At least when using a stapler,

Fig. 11.3 Gastrojejunostomy. Side-to-side anastomosis as functional end-to-side anastomosis using a stapler-cutter

Fig. 11.4 Gastrojejunostomy. Advancing a 12 mm calibration tube to avoid anastomotic stenosis

Fig. 11.5 Gastrojejunostomy. Suturing of the anterior wall

the calibration tube must be advanced before the stapler is released to ensure a sufficient width of the anastomosis. Due to the length of the gastric pouch, the formation of a tension-free anastomosis is achieved. Therefore, splitting the omentum majus is usually not necessary. The authors favour additional Kappeler sutures to achieve that the afferent loop remains significantly higher than the efferent loop.

Finally, the omentum is placed between the pouch and the remaining stomach. As in other procedures, placement of a drainage is optional, but is recommended by the authors for 1–3 days. Internal hernias through the Petersen's cleft are extremely rare even without closure of the cleft.

11.7 Omega-Loop Bypass as a Redo Procedure After Sleeve Gastrectomy

After releasing the predominantly minor adhesions at the antrum-corpus boundary, a retrogastric tunnel is created and the gastric sleeve is cut through with a stapler-cutter (◘ Fig. 11.6). Staple line reinforcement is optional.

11.8 Pitfalls

- No combination of maximum restriction and malabsorption: the gastric pouch should not be formed too narrowly.
- Pouch formation without calibration tube: A tube is considered obligatory analogous to sleeve gastrectomy. Otherwise, stenoses or fundus "diverticula" are inevitable.
- No gastric tube during pouch formation or anastomosis formation: Apart from the calibration tube, neither gastric nor temperature tubes should be placed in the esophagus. They can be inadvertently pushed forward into the stomach and extend into the staple sutures, leading to avoidable complications.
- Too much lateral tension on the gastric body or fundus can quickly lead to severe stenoses within the gastric sleeve.
- In order to prevent jejunogastric bile reflux, for formation of the gastrojejunostomy additional sutures according to Kappeler should be attached at a slight angle on the side of the afferent loop or a side-to-side anastomosis should be applied in the first place (◘ Fig. 11.2b).
- In case of perioperative nausea, a gastric tube should never be placed (risk of staple line suture perforation).

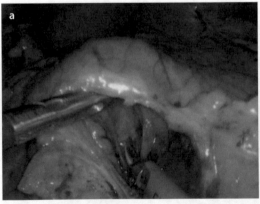
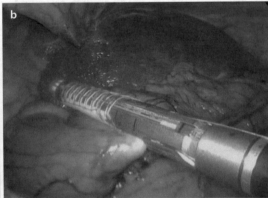

◘ **Fig. 11.6   a, b** Conversion of gastric sleeve into minigastric bypass. **a** Mobilisation and tunnelling of the gastric sleeve at the corpus-antrum boundary. **b** Cutting through the gastric sleeve at the corpus-antrum boundary with a stapler-cutter

- Special case "conversion of gastric sleeve—omega-loop bypass": Usually, this procedure is technically not complicated. Often, the gastric sleeve has to be mobilized only at the antrum-corpus boundary and released from adhesions. Subsequently, the same steps follow as in primary surgery with measurement of the small intestine and application of a side-to-side linear stapler anastomosis.

11.9 Peri- and Postoperative Management

The duration of the operation in experienced hands is less than 1 h, Rutledge himself states the duration to be 37 ± 34 min (Rutledge 2001). Similar to other obesity surgery and metabolic surgery procedures, the initial dietary regimen is standardised. In contrast to sleeve gastrectomy, fluids are tolerated very quickly when an omega-loop bypass is applied, as the physiological stenosis effect of the pylorus is bypassed.

The inpatient stay in the Rutledge series is 1.5 ± 1.6 days. Since the authors attach great importance to postoperative inpatient multidisciplinary support and training, outpatient or short inpatient stays are not recommended.

11.10 Results

In his long-term series of 2410 patients, Rutledge (2005) reports on a constant excess weight loss after 1 year of 80%. Less than 5% of patients regained more than 10 kg of weight in the following 4–5 years. In addition, an improvement of comorbidities is described with a high percentage for operated patients (GERD: 85%, diabetes: 83%, sleep apnea: 87%, hypertension: 80%, hypercholesterolemia: 89%, shortness of breath: 96%, urinary incontinence: 82%). In principle, the omega-loop bypass has a slightly stronger malabsorptive effect than the classical proximal Roux-en-Y gastric bypass.

Results of meta-analyses are also promising (■ Table 11.1).

Accordingly, the technically simpler omega-loop bypass appears superior to the classic proximal Roux-en-Y gastric bypass in terms of weight loss and diabetes control as well as in terms of learning curve, intra- and postoperative complications and long-term results. The latter seems to be more favourable only with regard to biliary reflux. Especially, high-risk patients (men, BMI > 50 kg/m^2, severe concomitant diseases) seem to benefit from MGB (review by Lee and Lin 2014). These findings are also supported by a prospective randomised study (Lee et al. 2005).

MGB patients are reported to have fewer abdominal symptoms postoperatively than Roux-en-Y gastric bypass patients with the same overall quality of life; they also have a higher stool frequency, which is why the Lee and Lin favour MGB especially for obese patients with constipation.

Compared to the sleeve gastrectomy, the MGB has the advantage of reversibility. Side effects of the "high pressure zone" gastric sleeve such as reflux and poor healing of leaks are also reduced.

11.11 Complications and Complication Management

Major complications occur on average with a frequency of 2%, half of which are due to leaks. The 30-day mortality rate is between 0% and 0.9% (review by Lee and Lin 2014). Under randomized conditions (Lee et al. 2005), MGB patients benefit from shorter surgery duration, less pain, shorter hospitalization and fewer postoperative complications compared to Roux-en-Y gastric bypass patients.

The rate of long-term complications is also low (Lee and Lin 2014). Only about 5% of those who have undergone surgery require conversion surgery, almost half of them due to severe malabsorption or insufficient weight loss (Lee et al. 2012). In these cases, the conversion into a gastric sleeve or a distal Roux-en-Y gastric bypass is recommended as redo operations.

Internal hernias are extremely rare, although they have to be considered in differential diagnosis of an acute abdomen in every gastric bypass surgery patient because of the high lethality. Even without mesenteric occlusion, the incidence of Petersen's hernia at 0.08% (Lee and Lin 2014) is 10–100 times lower than with Roux gastric bypass (>10% without, 1–2% with mesenteric occlusion) (Paroz et al. 2006). The reason for this is not exactly clear.

There is no evidence for a suspected increased rate of gastric carcinoma due to biliary reflux. The majority of gastric carcinomas after Roux-en-Y gastric bypass was found in the residual stomach, after an one-anastomosis bypass only one occurrence of a gastric carcinoma has been reported to date, as well in the residual stomach (Lee and Lin 2014).

References

Carbajo M, García-Caballero M, Toledano M, et al (2005) One-anastomosis gastric bypass by laparoscopy: results of the first 209 patients. Obes Surg. 15:398–404

Carbajo MA, Luque-de-León E (2015) Mini-gastric bypass/one-anastomosis gastric bypass-Standardizing the name. Obes Surg 25:858–859

Chakhtoura G, Zinzindohoué F, Ghanem Y, Ruseykin I, Dutranoy JC, Chevallier JM (2008) Primary results of laparoscopic mini-gastric bypass in a French obesity-surgery specialized university hospital. Obes Surg 18:1130–1133

Clarke MG, Wong K, Pearless L, Booth M (2013) Laparoscopic silastic ring mini-gastric bypass: a single centre experience. Obes Surg 23:1852–1857

Darabi S, Talebpour M, Zeinoddini A, Heidari R (2013) Laparoscopic gastric plication versus mini-gastric bypass surgery in the treatment of morbid obesity: a randomized clinical trial. Surg Obes Relat Dis 9:914–919

Kular KS, Manchanda N, Rutledge R (2014) A 6-year experience with 1054 mini-gastric bypasses-first study from Indian subcontinent. Obes Surg 24:1430–1435

Lee WJ, Lin YH (2014) Single-anastomosis gastric bypass (SAGB): appraisal of clinical evidence. Obes Surg 24:1749–1756

Lee WJ, Yu PJ, Wang W, Chen TC, Wei PL, Huang MT (2005) Laparoscopic Roux-en-Y versus mini-gastric bypass for the treatment of morbid obesity: a prospective randomized controlled clinical trial. Ann Surg 242:20–28

Lee WJ, Ser KH, Lee YC, Tsou JJ, Chen SC, Chen JC (2012) Laparoscopic Roux-en-Y vs. mini-gastric bypass for the treatment of morbid obesity: a 10-year experience. Obes Surg 22:1827–1834

Musella M, Susa A, Greco F et al (2013) The laparoscopic mini-gastric bypass: the Italian experience: outcomes from 974 consecutive cases in a multicenter review. Surg Endosc 28:156–163

Noun R, Skaff J, Riachi E, Daher R, Antoun NA, Nasr M (2012) One thousand consecutive mini-gastric bypass: short- and long-term outcome. Obes Surg 22:697–703

Paroz A, Calmes JM, Giusti V, Suter M (2006) Internal hernia after laparoscopic Roux-en-Y gastric bypass for morbid obesity: a continuous challenge in bariatric surgery. Obes Surg 16:1482–1487

Peraglie C (2008) Laparoscopic mini-gastric bypass (LMGB) in the super-super obese: outcomes in 16 patients. Obes Surg 18:1126–1129

Runkel N, Colombo-Benkmann M, Hüttl TP et al (2011) Evidence-based German guidelines for surgery for obesity. Int J Color Dis 26:397–404

Rutledge R (2001) The mini-gastric bypass: experience with the first 1274 cases. Obes Surg 11:276–280

Rutledge R, Walsh TR (2005) Continued results with mini-gastric bypass: six-year study in 2410 patients. Obes Surg 15:1304–1308

Further Readings

Lee WJ, Lee YC, Ser KH, Chen SC, Chen JC, Su YH (2010) Revisional surgery for laparoscopic minigastric bypass. Surg Obes Relat Dis 7:486–491

Rutledge RH (1973) Retroanastomotic hernias after gastrojejunal anastomoses. Ann Surg 77:547–553

Rutledge R (2014) Naming the mini-gastric bypass. Obes Surg 24:2173

11

Biliopancreatic Diversion (Operation According to Scopinaro)

A. Dietrich

Contents

© Springer-Verlag GmbH Germany, part of Springer Nature 2022
J. Ordemann, U. Elbelt (eds.), *Obesity and Metabolic Surgery*,
https://doi.org/10.1007/978-3-662-63227-7_12

12.1 Introduction

Biliopancreatic diversion (BPD) was first described in 1979 by Nicola Scopinaro, at that time still as open surgery with resection of the residual stomach (Scopinaro et al. 1979).

This is a purely malabsorptive procedure. The reconstruction technique corresponds to that of Roux-en-Y gastric bypass. However, with BPD, in contrast to gastric bypass, the common channel is only 50 cm long (malabsorption) and the gastric pouch is significantly larger (■ Fig. 12.1).

Due to the massive malabsorption and the resulting complications, the intervention is controversially discussed. While it is performed in the country of origin, Italy, in a relevant number of cases, in Germany it is in fact of no importance. According to the German Quality Assurance Study, it was performed 14 times in 2014, 6 times as a primary intervention and 8 times as a conversion operation after failure of another procedure.

As an option for a planned conversion to a malabsorptive procedure, a sufficiently large stomach is a prerequisite for BPD, e.g., after gastric banding or even in the case of a very wide tubular stomach.

The pronounced malabsorption leads to sustained weight loss and remission of comorbidities.

12.2 Indication and Preparation for Surgery

The perioperative risk profile of BPD is similar to that of standard Roux-en-Y gastric bypass. The indications and contraindications for bariatric or metabolic interventions apply without restriction.

However, the potential long-term complications of malabsorption and its health consequences, as well as social and professional implications, need to be discussed in detail with the patient. Of all bariatric interventions, BPD is the one with the highest risk of malabsorption despite oral supplementation and a balanced diet. Possible fatty stools, diarrhoea or frequent flatulence can limit the quality of life and the professional or social life.

Adherence in terms of aftercare and supplementation is essential.

This procedure should be viewed critically in women of childbearing age who wish to have children.

12

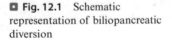

■ **Fig. 12.1** Schematic representation of biliopancreatic diversion

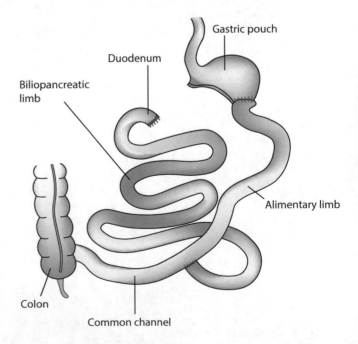

Under the following conditions a BPD may be considered:

- As a one-stage primary intervention if the patient so desires, accepting the long-term risks. To make or support this recommendation, a higher BMI and comorbidities such as type 2 diabetes mellitus should be present.
- After a sleeve gastrectomy with a relatively large tubular stomach in the case of
  - insufficient weight loss or weight regain,
  - persistent or recurrent type 2 diabetes (or other obesity-associated comorbidities)
- If the therapeutic goal is not achieved after horizontal gastroplasty or gastric banding.

The conversion to a BPD is also possible after Roux-en-Y gastric bypass. However, this operation is technically very complex and is therefore very rarely performed.

Under the following conditions, BPD should not be considered, or only to a limited extent

- In women of childbearing age with a desire to have children (increased risk of deficiency symptoms due to the high malabsorption).
- In patients with liver or biliary tract diseases where endoscopic access to the duodenum or papilla is necessary.
- A different procedure should be used for patients with certain professions, whose practice is not compatible with frequent bowel movements or flatulence.
- Where there are uncertainties regarding the absorption of drugs.

12.3 Surgical Technique

BPD can be performed as a primary intervention or as a conversion operation after another intervention has been performed. BPD is mainly performed as primary surgery.

The procedure should be performed laparoscopically. Open surgery is associated with increased complication rates and is not considered timely.

The surgical technique described below is based on the description by Nicola Scopinaro (Scopinaro et al. 2007).

🛈 Biliopancreatic diversion is a highly malabsorptive procedure. The restriction must not be too strong to ensure an adequate food supply.

12.3.1 Laparoscopy, Trocar Placement and Clarification of Operability

First of all, the pneumoperitoneum is created. The use of a non-cutting visual trocar can be considered a standard access. The risk of vascular or hollow organ injury must be taken into account, especially in the case of those who have been operated on previously. Further trocars should be inserted under visual control.

The first trocar (camera trocar) is inserted approximately 15–20 cm caudally of the xiphoid on the left paramedian side. Since the cut through the stomach and the gastroenterostomy are performed further distal in the stomach, the trocars should also be placed somewhat more caudally than in gastric bypass.

The following trocars are inserted as working trocars: For the operation in the upper abdomen, one 12-trocar each in the right and left upper abdomen and one 5-trocar in the left lateral middle abdomen. For the localization and measurement of the ileum as well as for the enteroenterostomy, one trocar of 5 is placed in the right lateral middle abdomen and one trocar of 12 in the left middle abdomen.

A preferably fixable liver retractor should be used to provide a clear view of the stomach by lifting the left liver lobe. In the case of rearrangements, care must be taken to ensure that no parenchymal tears occur in the often massively enlarged liver.

This is followed by an inspection of the abdomen and clarification of the operability. Besides the general operability, special attention must be paid to the mobility of the ileum:

The ileum must be freely movable over 250 cm measured aborally from the Bauhin's valve and must be able to be guided without tension to the planned anastomosis to the middle stomach.

When clarifying the mobility of the ileum, it is advisable to simultaneously measure the loops and apply the foot point anastomosis.

12.3.2 Transection of the Stomach

The first step is to determine the height of the planned incision of the stomach. This can be done horizontally or in a staircase. The volume of the stomach for food intake should be 200–500 ml.

At the ends of the planned incision line, the bursa omentalis is opened on the small or large curvature side close to the stomach wall and then the stomach is divided, usually with stapling devices.

The remaining stomach remains in situ as with the gastric bypass.

In the case of an increased bleeding tendency (e.g., when taking antiplatelet aggregation medication, intensified anticoagulation beyond thrombosis prophylaxis, etc.) the use of staple line reinforcement should be considered.

This part of the operation is performed in anti-Trendelenburg position, the surgeon stands between the patient's legs.

12.3.3 Measurement of the Loop Lengths

If not already done at the beginning when clarifying the operability, the measurement of the loop lengths for the reconstruction to restore the passage is done now. For this step it is advisable to change the surgeon to the left side of the patient, the operating table is placed horizontally. The coecum is sought out and the ileum is measured orally.

Measure 50 cm of the common channel and place a thread or colour mark (with directional mark) there. From there, the alimentary loop is measured orally to 200 cm. At this point, the intestine is then cut through with

a stapler. The oral end is led to the previously marked ileum (50 cm before the Bauhin's valve). This is where the side-to-side ileoileostomy is performed.

The biliopancreatic diversion is reconstructed classically according to Roux-en-Y with a common channel only 50 cm long.

12.3.4 Small Intestine Anastomosis

The anastomosis techniques vary, see foot point anastomosis for gastric bypass (▶ Sect. 10.7). A stapler anastomosis is possible as well as hand suturing. The anastomosis should be wide to prevent stenosis, e.g., due to subsequent scarring. To avoid an internal hernia, the mesenteric slit should be closed with a non-resorbable suture.

12.3.5 Gastroileostomy

To perform the gastroileostomy, it is recommended that the patient be repositioned in the anti-Trendelenburg position; the surgeon stands between the legs.

The severed ileum is usually led antecolically to the stomach. In order to avoid unnecessary traction on the anastomosis, the free part of the omentum majus can be split if necessary.

Different techniques can be used for anastomosis. Recommended are the complete hand suture or the use of linear staple suturing devices. Circular staplers should not be used if at all possible, as insertion of the stapler head into the ileum (lower lumen than the jejunum in gastric bypass) can be problematic.

Before closing the anastomosis, a stronger stomach tube (e.g. 28 Fr) should be pushed over the anastomosis under visual control in order to be able to check the tightness of the anastomosis with a blue sample after complete closure.

After checking the site and reconstruction, it is recommended to insert a drainage, usually to the gastroileostomy. A drainage should always be inserted if the transformation operation has been carried out, as in this case a higher fistula and bleeding rate can be assumed.

12.3.6 Simultaneous Appendectomy, Cholecystectomy and Hiatus Hernias

Due to the intraoperative manipulations in the right lower abdomen (measurement of the small intestine aborally of the Bauhin's valve) and the position of the foot point anastomosis there, unspecific pain (adhesion problems etc.) may occur in the right lower abdomen. To avoid differential diagnostic problems with appendicitis, some surgeons perform a simultaneous appendectomy. There is no evidence or general recommendation for this.

As a result of the rapid weight loss after bariatric surgery that occurs after BPD—and here also an increased reabsorption of bile acids through the long biliopancreatic loop—the risk of gallstone formation is increased in those affected. It can be reduced by prophylactic administration of ursodeoxycholic acid.

As an alternative, some surgeons generally perform a cholecystectomy even if there is no evidence of stones. The reasons for this are the risk of gallstone formation, the non-existent option of endoscopic retrograde cholangiopancreaticography (ERCP) in the case of stone loss and the fact that a later cholecystectomy is then potentially more technically complex due to adhesions. There is also no evidence or general recommendation for this. However, in the presence of cholecystolithiasis—especially symptomatic—a cholecystectomy should always be performed simultaneously.

The hiatus oesophagei should be inspected and a hernia, if present, should be closed.

12.4 Pitfalls

- The indication for BPD must be accompanied by a detailed patient education, in which it is pointed out that BPD is not a regulatory intervention.
- The pronounced malabsorption is very effective in terms of weight control and remission of obesity-associated comorbidities. However, despite consistent substitution, deficiency symptoms and frequent diarrhoea or fatty stools can occur.

> **Practical Tip**
>
> Biliopancreatic diversion should only be performed in centers with appropriate expertise. Very consistent, lifelong follow-up care is obligatory.

- While there is a certain variability in the stomach volume or the length of the alimentary canal, the measurement of the common channel must be exact. In order to avoid cachexia and disproportionate malabsorption, the common channel must not be shorter than 50 cm; a longer length would result in an increased intake of nutrients or energy sources.
- The restriction caused by the reduced stomach and gastroileostomy must not be too strong.

12.5 Results

BPD offers excellent results with an excess weight loss (EWL) of up to 75%, which is long-term stable due to malabsorption (Scopinaro et al. 2007). Remission rates of type 2 diabetes, even with preoperative insulin therapy are reported to be up to 100%, in meta-analyses they are 89% (Scopinaro et al. 2007; Panunzi et al. 2015).

Compared to the so-called "gold standard" gastric bypass, the short and medium-term results (2-year results from a prospective randomized study in type 2 diabetics) are equivalent with regard to EWL; however, the remission rate of type 2 diabetes is higher after BPD (Mingrone et al. 2012). In the long run, BPD is more effective also with respect to EWL due to the high malabsorption.

After the procedure, high remission rates can also be expected for other obesity-associated comorbidities—such as arterial hypertension, sleep apnoea syndrome, steatosis hepatis, dyslipidemia, etc.

Comparing classical BPD with bilio-pancreatic diversion with Duodenal Switch (BPD-DS), equivalent results are shown with regard to weight reduction and influence on obesity-associated comorbidities. BPD-DS, however, is associated with a more complex surgical technique and consequently with higher perioperative morbidity and mortality compared to classic BPD according to Scopinaro (▶ Chap. 13). The risk of dumping, which exists after BPD, is not increased in BPD-DS due to the preserved passage over the pylorus. Due to the shorter common channel, malabsorption is higher in BPD due to the procedure.

Even if rarely reported, there may be excessive weight loss. In this case a supplementary diet should be administered. If surgical correction is considered, an extension of the common channel in favour of the biliopancreatic loop is recommended.

12.6 Morbidity and Mortality

The morbidity and mortality of BPD is similar to that of Roux-en-Y gastric bypass. The procedure is considered safe. Severe complications such as anastomosis insufficiency, (post-)bleeding or abscess formation rarely occur.

The general rules of visceral surgery apply to complication management. Due to the limited reserves of patients, aggressive complication management must be carried out without delay. The indication for relaparoscopy must be generously provided. In addition, promising endoscopic methods (e.g., stent or vacuum treatment) and interventional radiological methods (e.g., CT-supported drainage of an abscess) must be used to avoid revision surgery if possible.

Postoperatively the serum myoglobin should be checked. With an increased BMI and long surgery time, the risk of muscular damage increases due to the long period of lying in relaxation, which in extreme cases can lead to kidney damage. In the case of increased myoglobin levels, an appropriate fluid intake must be made.

In the case of transformation operations, attention must be paid to the risks of vascular or hollow organ injury when the pneumoperitoneum is applied or—in the case of a second operation—during adhesiolysis.

In case of gastroileal or ileoileal anastomosis insufficiency or post-operative bleeding, an urgent relaparoscopy and revision should be performed. Depending on the findings, gastroileostomy can also be performed gastroscopically using a stent, clip or vacuum; preferably if a local target drainage is still present.

After BPD, the substitution should be done with special preparations, such as those available for post gastric bypass conditions, but this is often not sufficient. Commercially available multivitamin tablets from discounters are not recommended.

Despite consistent supplementation, deficiency symptoms occur after this malabsorptive procedure in over 90% of cases, and there are no differences to BPD-DS (Homan et al. 2015). Due to the procedure-related malabsorption as well as further unbalanced nutrition, the following deficiencies are the most common: hypoalbumin or hypoproteinemia, iron deficiency (with anaemia), deficiency of fat-soluble vitamins (ADEK) as well as of vitamins B_1, B_6, B_{12}, deficiency of zinc, copper and magnesium (Homan et al. 2015). This can cause corresponding neurological (vitamin B deficiency), dermatological (vitamin A or zinc deficiency), hematological (iron or vitamin B_{12} deficiency) or other symptoms.

In addition to the prophylactic intake of the above vitamins and trace elements, it is particularly important to ensure that calcium is administered as citrate with sufficient vitamin D (otherwise there is hardly any absorption) and that the protein intake and drinking quantity are adequate (Homan et al. 2015).

Other known complications after BPD are: gallstone formation, kidney stone formation and secondary hyperparathyroidism.

Biliopancreatic diversion leads to deficiency symptoms in a high percentage of patients despite routine supplementation. Consistent follow-up with laboratory controls and appropriate substitution are necessary.

In particular, a high rate of anastomosis ulcers is to be expected postoperatively, especially in the case of alcohol or nicotine history, which is why routine administration of proton pump inhibitors is recommended for up to 18 months postoperatively (Weiner 2006).

Due to (severe) long-term complications, conversion surgery or reverse surgery is necessary in 3–18% of cases (Topart and Becouarn 2015).

References

Homan S, Betzel B, Aarts EO, Dogan K et al (2015) Vitamin and mineral deficiencies after biliopancreatic diversion and biliopancreatic diversion with duodenal switch—the rule rather than the exception. Obes Surg 25:1626–1632

Mingrone G, Panunzi S, De Gaetano A et al (2012) Bariatric surgery versus conventional medical therapy for type 2 diabetes. N Engl J Med 366:1577–1585

Panunzi S, De Gaetano A, Carnicelli A, Mingrone G (2015) Predictors of remission of diabetes mellitus in severely obese individuals undergoing bariatric surgery: do BMI or procedure choice matter? A meta-analysis. Ann Surg 261:459–467

Scopinaro N, Gianetta E, Civalleri D, Bonalumi U, Bachi V (1979) Bilio-pancreatic bypass for obesity: II. Initial experience in man. Br J Surg 66:618–620

Scopinaro N, Marinari G, Camerini C, Papadia F (2007) Biliopancreatic diversion: physiological and metabolic aspects. In: Parini U, Nebiolo PE (eds) Bariatric surgery multidisciplinary approach and surgical techniques, 2nd edn. Musumeci Editore, pp 314–342

Topart PA, Becouarn G (2015) Revision and reversal after biliopancreatic diversion for excessive side effects or ineffective weight loss: a review of the current literature on indications and procedures. Surg Obes Relat Dis 11:965–972

Weiner R (2006) Adipositaschirurgie—Indikation und Therapieverfahren, 1. Aufl. 2006. UNI-MED, Bremen, S95–99

Further Reading

Stein J, Stier C, Raab H, Weiner R (2014) Review article: the nutritional and pharmacological consequences of obesity surgery. Aliment Pharmacol Ther 40: 582–609

Biliopancreatic Diversion with Duodenal Switch

A. Dietrich

Contents

© Springer-Verlag GmbH Germany, part of Springer Nature 2022
J. Ordemann, U. Elbelt (eds.), *Obesity and Metabolic Surgery*,
https://doi.org/10.1007/978-3-662-63227-7_13

BPD-DS was first performed on obese patients in 1988 by Douglas Hess, initially as an open surgery (Hess and Hess 1998). Due to the good results, the procedure became established and was then performed laparoscopically by Michael Gagner before the turn of the millennium (Ren et al. 2000).

13.1 Specific Indications for BPD-DS

In view of the increased risk profile compared to standard interventions, a detailed discussion of the risk-benefit balance must be held with the patient. The indications and contraindications for bariatric or metabolic interventions apply without restriction.

Under the following conditions a BPD-DS can be considered:

- As a one-stage primary intervention if the patient so desires, while accepting the risks. To make or support this recommendation, a higher BMI (>50 kg/m²) and comorbidities such as type 2 diabetes mellitus should be present.
- After sleeve gastrectomy in the case of:
  - insufficient weight loss or weight regain,
  - persistent or recurrent type 2 diabetes (or other obesity-associated comorbidities)
- After Roux-en-Y gastric bypass (or bypasses without preserved pyloric passage) with therapy-resistant dumping
- If the therapeutic goal is not achieved after bypass or gastric band surgery (see point 2, sleeve gastrectomy), provided that a corresponding reconstruction is technically possible).

Under certain conditions, a BDP-DS should not be considered or only be considered to a limited extent:

- Patients with severe concomitant diseases (renal insufficiency, liver diseases), as the already increased perioperative morbidity and mortality then increases further.
- Women of childbearing age with a desire to have children (increased risk of deficiency symptoms due to the high malabsorption).

- In case of existing severe reflux disease, primarily another bariatric procedure should be considered (preferably Roux-en-Y gastric bypass), because sleeve gastrectomy can lead to a worsening of a pre-existing reflux. However, the data on this is inconsistent.
- For patients from certain occupational groups for whom frequent stool discharge or flatulence is unacceptable, a different procedure should be chosen.

13.2 Surgical Technique

The BPD-DS can primarily be carried out in one or two stages. First, a sleeve gastrectomy should be performed and the result awaited. If the therapy goal is not achieved (▶ Sect. 13.1), a conversion operation, in this case the duodenal switch, can be performed. The principle of the operation is shown schematically in ◻ Fig. 13.1. For a large number of patients, the second step will no longer be necessary or not desired by them. Both operations are performed laparoscopically.

> **Practical Tip**
>
> A two-stage procedure should be favoured, the first step being a sleeve gastrectomy.

Among others, Ren et al. were able to show that a two-stage procedure (first sleeve gastrectomy and then, after weight reduction, duodenal switch) resulted in significantly fewer complications overall (8% vs. 38%) (Ren et al. 2000).

With a BMI < 50 kg/m², a one-stage procedure is also possible if patients do not wish to wait for the therapeutic result of an initially performed single sleeve gastrectomy or if, for example, diabetes mellitus type 2 exists with the need for very high insulin doses.

In older studies it was shown that patients with a BMI > 60 kg/m² and BPD-DS had a mortality or morbidity rate of 6.5% and 23% respectively, which is unacceptable today, if the procedure is performed in one stage; how-

◘ Fig. 13.1 Schematic representation of biliopancreatic diversion with duodenal switch

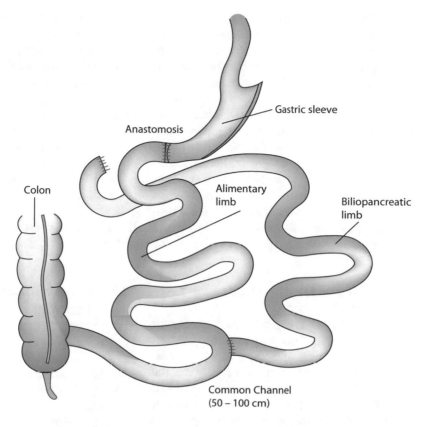

Gastric sleeve

Anastomosis

Colon

Alimentary limb

Biliopancreatic limb

Common Channel (50 – 100 cm)

ever, the learning curve and partially open surgical techniques certainly played a role at that time (Manger et al. 2009). Specialised centres with high case numbers—of which there are, however, only a few—also report case series with one-stage procedures in the higher BMI range without mortality and complication rates of 14.4% (Buchwald et al. 2008).

13.2.1 Laparoscopy, Trocar Placement and Clarification of Operability

First of all, the pneumoperitoneum is created. The use of a non-cutting visual trocar can be considered a standard access. The risk of vascular or hollow organ injury must be taken into account, especially in the case of those who have been operated on previously. Further trocars should be inserted under visual control.

The first trocar (camera trocar) is inserted approximately 15 cm caudally of the xiphoid on the left paramedian side. For sleeve gastrectomy a 12 trocar each in the right and left upper abdomen and a 5 trocar in the left lateral middle abdomen follow. For the duodenal switch, an additional 5 trocar is placed in the right lateral middle abdomen and a 12 trocar in the left middle abdomen.

A preferably fixable liver retractor should be used to ensure adequate visibility during the individual surgical steps. In the case of rearrangements, care must be taken to ensure that no parenchymal tears occur in the often massively enlarged liver.

This is followed by an inspection of the abdomen and clarification of the operability. This must include:

– Possibility of sleeve gastrectomy or sleeve reduction by far sleeve;
– Option of the duodenal switch:
  – The duodenum must be safely dissectable (exclusion of adhesions in the right upper abdomen after cholecystectomy, pancreatitis, etc.)

– The ileum, measured backwards from the Bauhin's valve, must be freely movable over 250 cm and must be able to be guided without tension to the planned anastomosis at the duodenum.

Regardless of the procedure (whether a one- or two-stage procedure), sleeve gastrectomy or sleeve reduction should be performed first. Once the operability of the duodenal switch has been clarified, the preparation of the duodenum or small intestine can be started. When clarifying the mobility of the ileum, it is advisable to simultaneously measure the loops and apply the foot point anastomosis.

13.2.2 Sleeve Gastrectomy

The first step is the sleeve gastrectomy or sleeve reduction. This part of the operation is performed in an anti-Trendelenburg position, with the surgeon standing between the patient's legs. The left lobe of the liver must be lifted with the help of the liver retractor. As with all bariatric operations, the presence of a hiatus hernia must be ruled out. In principle, the principles described in ▶ Chap. 9 for sleeve gastrectomy apply; however, in the case of a single-stage procedure, with the deviation that the gastric sleeve should be applied more widely, since the combination of severe malabsorption with excessive restriction must be avoided.

The following aspects are essential for sleeve gastrectomy:

— A mobilization of the fundus up to the angle of His on the large-curvature side is necessary to achieve a complete fundus resection. Only in this way can a reduction of the so-called hunger hormone ghrelin be achieved. The dissection is usually performed with sealing and severing laparoscopic instruments.

— The sleeve gastrectomy begins about 3–5 cm prepyloric. In this way the pumping function of the antrum can be maintained and gastric emptying disorders can be avoided.

— The use of a 34- to 60-Fr bougie is recommended for tubular stomach formation.

For the single-stage procedure, a rather further bougie should be used. Stapling instruments are usually used to form a tube stomach; the thickness of the staple is reduced from the antrum to the angle of His.

— In the case of an increased bleeding tendency (e.g., when taking antiplatelet aggregation medication, intensified anticoagulation beyond thrombosis prophylaxis, etc.) the use of staple boosters should be considered.

If a one-stage procedure is desired, the ileum is then measured.

13.2.3 Measurement of Loop Lengths

For this step it is advisable to change the surgeon to the left side of the patient. The coecum is visited and the ileum is measured aborally. 75–100 cm of the common channel is measured and a suture or color marker (with directional marker) is applied. From this marker the alimentary loop is measured orally to 150 cm. Here the intestine is then cut through with a stapler. The oral end is led to the previously marked ileum and then the side-to-side ileoileostomy is applied.

As an alternative to Roux-en-Y reconstruction, a single loop reconstruction is also possible (Single Anastomosis Duodenoileal Bypass with Sleeve Gastrectomy, SADI-S). For this purpose, the ileum is measured to 250 cm from the Bauhin's valve and then the duodenoileostomy is performed there using the technique described above (Sánchez-Pernaute et al. 2015).

13.2.4 Small Intestine Anastomosis (In Case of Classical Reconstruction According to Roux-en-Y)

The anastomosis techniques vary, see foot point anastomosis for gastric bypass (▶ Chap. 10). Forklift anastomosis is possible as well as hand suturing. The anastomosis should be wide in order to prevent stenosis, e.g., due to later scarring. To avoid an internal hernia, the mesenteric slit should be closed with a non-resorbable suture.

13.2.5 Duodenum Transection

This step can also be performed before measuring the small intestinal loops, once the operability has been clarified. It represents the so-called "point of no return"; a re-anastomosis of the duodenum is difficult and risky.

As in cholecystectomy, the patient is in the anti-Trendelenburg position, possibly tilted slightly to the left, with the surgeon standing between his legs.

The liver retractor should be used to allow a clear view of the liver hilus.

The duodenum is cut approximately 2–3 cm distal to the pylorus, right lateral to the hepatoduodenal ligament (□ Fig. 13.2). In order to avoid injuries of the pylorus—cutting through the pylorus increases the risk of dumping—and of the pancreatic head—with the risk of fistulation—extremely subtle preparations should be made. The peritoneum is then opened at the upper and lower edge of the duodenum, the latter is then tunnelled under near the intestinal wall.

If sealing systems are used, thermal damage to the duodenal wall or pancreas must be taken into account. Careful preparation and

hemostasis is indicated, all surrounding vessels are preserved.

If the post-pyloric duodenum is circumferentially prepared, it is recommended to loop it with a tape and then cut it with a linear stapler (the authors use a closed staple thickness of 1 mm).

❗ Special care is required when preparing near the pancreatic head. Pancreatic fistulas, bleeding or a duodenal stump insufficiency are potentially serious complications.

13.2.6 Duodenoileostomy

The aboral jejunum loop is guided towards the liver hilus and fixed with a holding suture. In order to enable a tension-free anastomosis, a splitting of the omentum is recommended. Various techniques can be used to create an anastomosis (hand suture, use of a linear or circular stapler). The most common is the double-row continuous hand suture. The first step is the continuous suture of the back wall (the authors use 2-0-Vicryl for the anastomoses in laparoscopic bariatric surgery). Then both lumina are opened over a distance of about 1.5–2 cm (□ Fig. 13.3), the back wall is secured with a second row of sutures (□ Fig. 13.4). Usually, a stomach tube (28 Fr) is then pushed over the anastomosis under visual control and the front wall is then sutured in two consecutive rows. The tightness of the anastomosis should be checked with a blue sample.

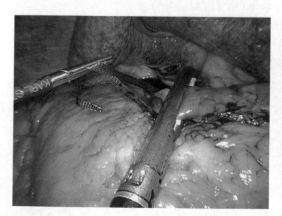

□ **Fig. 13.2** Looping and severing of the postpyloric duodenum

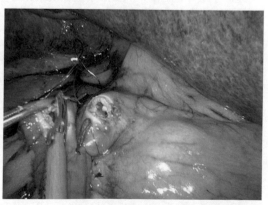

□ **Fig. 13.3** Opening of the intestinal lumens after the first row of sutures on the back wall

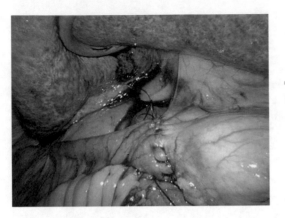

⬛ Fig. 13.4 Completed end-to-side duodenojejunostomy (two-row continuous hand suture)

13.2.7 Simultaneous Appendectomy and Cholecystectomy

Recommendations for simultaneous appendectomy and cholecystectomy are detailed in ▶ Sect. 12.3.6.

13.3 Pitfalls

- A detailed patient information must be provided with the indication for BPD-DS. It must be clear to all involved that BPD-DS is on the one hand the most effective bariatric and metabolic surgery, but on the other hand is associated with a significantly higher perioperative morbidity and mortality.
- The risk of patients developing deficiency symptoms or suffering from frequent diarrhoea or fatty stools in the long term, even with consistent substitution, should not be underestimated. Only an appropriately experienced interdisciplinary team (surgery, internal medicine, psychosomatic medicine and nutritional therapy) can successfully care for these patients.
- Duodenal switch surgery should only be performed in centers with appropriate expertise. As with all bariatric procedures, the indication should be interdisciplinary.
- In order to avoid cachexia, the restriction must not be too strong in view of the mal-

absorption due to the short common channel, i.e. the tubular stomach should be somewhat wider, even if there are no clear guidelines here.
- Due to the nature of the procedure, BPD-DS involves additional risks due to the preparation next to the pancreatic head, the duodenal stump and the duodenoileostomy, which is usually performed by hand suture. The expertise of surgeons experienced in laparoscopy is required to avoid a learning curve.

13.4 Results

BPD-DS offers excellent long-term results with an excess weight loss (EWL) of up to 80% and remission rates of type 2 diabetes of up to almost 100% (depending on the duration and severity of the pre-existing type 2 diabetes) (Gagner and Gumps 2007; Gumps et al. 2007; Kim et al. 2003; Prachand et al. 2006; Risstad et al. 2015; Weiner 2010).

High remission rates are also expected for other obesity-related co-morbidities such as arterial hypertension, sleep apnea syndrome, steatosis hepatis, dyslipidemia, etc.

Comparing the results with the gold standard of bariatric surgery, Roux-en-Y gastric bypass, Hedberg et al. were able to show in a meta-analysis that BPD-DS leads to an additional weight loss of an average of 6.2 BMI points. The remission rate of type 2 diabetes is 88% vs. 76% for Roux-en-Y gastric bypass (Hedberg et al. 2014).

With regard to the results—weight reduction and influence on obesity-associated co-morbidities—the more complex surgical technique of BPD-DS is roughly equivalent to the classic BPD according to Scopinaro, but with the advantage that the risk of dumping is lower due to the pylorus preservation and also the risk of severe malabsorption (with diarrhoea) is reduced due to the longer common channel.

If only slight weight loss or incomplete remission of co-morbidities occurs in the postoperative course, this is usually due to insufficient restriction (sleeve dilatation), incorrect eating habits or inadequate physical activity.

Regarding excessive weight loss, please refer to ▶ Chap. 12.

13.5 Morbidity and Mortality

Compared to the most common bariatric procedures (sleeve gastrectomy and Roux-en-Y gastric bypass), BPD-DS is associated with significantly increased perioperative morbidity and mortality. In the literature, complication rates of up to 38% for a single-stage procedure (Ren et al. 2000) and up to 30% for a two-stage procedure (Silecchia et al. 2009) have been reported, although these are partly due to the learning curve.

The most frequent complications are, as with the other bariatric procedures, fistulas of the staple suture, anastomotic insufficiencies, abscesses or (post-) bleeding.

Duodenal switch is accompanied by complications such as pancreatic fistulas or truncated duodenal insufficiency due to the preparation at the pancreatic head and the cutting of the duodenum; especially the latter is associated with high mortality. If a duodenal truncation insufficiency is suspected, if it is fresh, it should be reapplied and, if necessary, a T-drain system should be installed to reduce the secretion load. In the case of chronic fistulas, targeted drainage is often the only option.

With regard to complication management, reference is made to the recommendations in ▶ Chap. 12.

In the case of a two-stage procedure, attention must be paid to the risks of vascular or hollow organ injury when the pneumoperitoneum is applied or—in the case of a second procedure—during adhesiolysis.

In the case of duodenodenal or ileoileal anastomosis insufficiency or post-bleeding, an urgent relaparoscopy and revision should be performed. Duodenoileostomy can also be performed gastroscopically with a stent, clip or vacuum; preferably if a local target drainage is still present.

In the long-term course, the reoperation rates according to BPD-DS are compara-tively low. Strong attention must be paid to deficiency symptoms, which can occur in over 90% of cases despite substitution (Homan et al. 2015). According to BPD-DS, substitution should be carried out with special preparations such as those available for conditions following gastric bypass. Commercially available multivitamin tablets from discounters are not recommended.

Please refer to ▶ Chap. 12 for recommendations on how to avoid deficiencies and complications.

> **Practical Tip**
>
> Since the duodenal switch can often lead to deficiency symptoms due to its pronounced malabsorption, consistent substitution and aftercare is required especially in these patients, which also requires appropriate compliance.

References

Buchwald H, Oien DM (2013) Metabolic/bariatric surgery worldwide 2011. Obes Surg 23:427–436

Buchwald H, Kellogg TA, Leslie DB, Ikramuddin S (2008) Duodenal switch operative mortality and morbidity are not impacted by body-mass-index. Ann Surg 248:541–548

Gagner M, Gumbs AA (2007) Gastric banding: conversion to sleeve, bypass, or DS. Surg Endosc 21:1931–1935

Gumbs AA, Pomp A, Gagner M (2007) Revisional bariatric surgery for inadequate weight loss. Obes Surg 17:1137–1145

Hedberg J, Sundström J, Sundbom M (2014) Duodenal switch versus Roux-en-Y gastric bypass for morbid obesity: systematic review and meta-analysis of weight results, diabetes resolution and early complications in single-centre comparisons. Obes Rev 15:555–563

Hess DS, Hess DW (1998) Biliopancreatic diversion with a duodenal switch. Obes Surg 8:267–282

Homan S, Betzel B, Aarts EO et al (2015) Vitamin and mineral deficiencies after biliopancreatic diversion and biliopancreatic diversion with duodenal switch—the rule rather than the exception. Obes Surg 25:1626–1632

Kim WW, Gagner M, Kini S, Inabnet WB, Quinn T, Herron D, Pomp A (2003) Laparoscopic vs. open biliopancreatic diversion with duodenal switch: a comparative study. J Gastrointest Surg 7:552–557

Manger T, Hohmann U, Stroh C (2009) Surgical technique and outcome in metabolic and bariatric surgery: biliopancreatic diversion. Zentralbl Chir 134:38–42

Prachand VN, Davee RT, Alverdy JC (2006) Duodenal switch provides superior weight loss in the super-obese (BMI $\geq$ 50 kg/m^2) compared with gastric bypass. Ann Surg 244:611–619

Ren CJ, Patterson E, Gagner M (2000) Early results of laparoscopic biliopancreatic diversion with duodenal switch: a case series of 40 consecutive patients. Obes Surg 10:514–523

Risstad H, Søvik TT, Engström M et al (2015) Five-year outcomes after laparoscopic gastric bypass and laparoscopic duodenal switch in patients with body-mass-index of 50–60: a randomized clinical trial. JAMA Surg 150:352–361

Sánchez-Pernaute A, Rubio MÁ, Conde M, Arrue E, Pérez-Aguirre E, Torres A (2015) Single-anastomosis duodenoileal bypass as a second step after sleeve gastrectomy. Surg Obes Relat Dis 11:351–355

Silecchia G, Rizzello M, Casella G, Fioriti M, Soricelli E, Basso N (2009) Two-stage laparoscopic biliopancreatic diversion with duodenal switch as treatment of high-risk super-obese patients: analysis of complications. Surg Endosc 23:1032–1037

Weiner R (2010) Indications and principles of metabolic surgery. Chirurg 81:379–395

Further Readings

Aasprang A, Andersen JR, Våge V, Kolotkin RI, Natvig GK (2013) Five-year changes in health-related quality of life after biliopancreatic diversion with duodenal switch. Obes Surg 23:1662–1668

Iannelli A, Schneck AS, Dahman M, Negri C, Gugenheim J (2009) Two-step laparoscopic duodenal switch for superobesity: a feasibility study. Surg Endosc 23:2385–2389

Stein J, Stier C, Raab H, Weiner R (2014) Review article: the nutritional and pharmacological consequences of obesity surgery. Aliment Pharmacol Ther 40:582–609

Weiner R, Blanco-Engert R, Weiner S, Pomhoff I, Schramm M (2004) Laparoscopic biliopancreatic diversion with duodenal switch: three different duodeno-ileal anastomotic techniques and initial experience. Obes Surg 14:334–340

Postoperative Management of Bariatric Surgery Patients

H. Berger, J. Ordemann, U. Elbelt, T. Hofmann, and C. Menenakos

Contents

© Springer-Verlag GmbH Germany, part of Springer Nature 2022
J. Ordemann, U. Elbelt (eds.), *Obesity and Metabolic Surgery*,
https://doi.org/10.1007/978-3-662-63227-7_14

14.1 Initial Diet Regimen After Bariatric Surgery

H. Berger

Due to the altered anatomy of the gastrointestinal tract, patients may experience postoperative changes in nutrient intake and eating habits. Postoperative nutritional management aims to optimise nutrient intake, to monitor eating behaviour and to prevent nutrient deficiency symptoms and diseases by supplementation.

Diet regimen after bariatric surgery ensures the supply of energy and nutrients to patients while minimizing nutrition-related complaints during the healing process. The post-operative diet regimen consists of three stages. The duration of each stage depends on the specific operation performed and the individual recovery (Dieckmann 2013).

14.1.1 First Stage

In the first and second postoperative week it is recommended to offer liquid food. On the first and second day after the operation, only small amounts of liquids should be drunk, i.e., sips of unsweetened tea and non-carbonated water. If these quantities are well tolerated, the fluid intake can be increased and broth can be added (Dieckmann 2013). If well tolerated, the patient can be given protein-containing meals from the third day onwards, such as unsweetened milk or natural yoghurt dishes as well as protein supplements. In addition, finely pureed vegetable soups, mashed potatoes and finely pureed fruit, such as banana and apple, are usually well tolerated by patients. Due to the low stomach volume after the procedure,

4–6 meals per day are recommended, whereby a meal volume of 100–200 ml should not be exceeded during the first stage (Hellbardt 2013). To achieve an early feeling of satiety, it is recommended to separate eating and drinking. The following overview gives the eating behaviour rules after bariatric interventions for all time periods modified according to Moizé et al. (2010).

Eating Behaviour Rules After Bariatric Interventions (Mod. According to Moizé et al. 2010)

- 5–6 meals, 3 main meals and 2–3 snacks per day
- Avoidance of carbonated drinks
- Chew your food properly, eat in small bites
- Portion small quantities onto the plate
- Eat consciously, consider the feeling of satiety
- Eat slowly, allow at least 20 min
- Separate drinking and eating, drink 30 min before and only again 30 min after eating
- Take daily vitamin and mineral supplements and protein supplements if necessary

---

14.1.2 Second Stage

The second stage of the dietary regimen aims at the transition from liquid food to soft food. In the second to fourth postoperative week, the patient is offered pureed or soft meals. Depending on the patient's tolerance, slowly more solid foods (◼ Table 14.1) are added to the diet. A high-protein, low-fat and low-sugar diet is the basis for the choice of food.

◻ Table 14.1 Exemplary food selection of pureed and soft foods (2–4 weeks after bariatric surgery)

Food group	Food examples
Beverages	Non-carbonated water, unsweetened tea
Fruit and vegetables	Bananas, apples (low acidity varieties), pears carrots, zucchini, broccoli, other non-flatulent vegetables (initially better tolerated: steamed or pureed)
Cereals (products) and potatoes	Toast, rusk, cereal products made from wheat, maize, oats, e.g. flour, starch or semolina, boiled potatoes, mashed potatoes (lactose-free if necessary)
Milk and dairy products	Low-fat variants of milk, natural yoghurt, quark, cheese (maximum 30% in dry matter), (lactose-free if necessary)
Meat, fish, egg and sausages	Lean meat: veal, chicken Egg, prepared low-fat Lean sausage: cooked ham (without fat rim), poultry sausage
Fats and oils	Vegetable oils, e.g. rapeseed oil, margarine
Spices	No pungent spices

◻ Table 14.2 Foods that can cause complaints after bariatric surgery

Food group	Food examples
Beverages	Coffee, alcohol, sugary and carbonated drinks
Fruit and vegetables	Pineapple, bananas, rhubarb Mushrooms, asparagus, cabbage, green beans
Cereals (products) and potatoes	White bread, rusk, noodles, rice, fried products
Milk and dairy products	Milk, high-fat dairy products
Meat, fish, egg and sausages	Beef, seafood, raw ham
Food rich in fat and sugar	Sweets, fried food, etc.

14.1.3 Third Stage

The third stage is the transition from pureed or soft food to light diet. From the fourth postoperative week onwards, if the previous diet is well tolerated, more solid foods can be carefully added to the diet. The third stage is therefore the transition to long-term nutrition after bariatric surgery (see also ▶ Sect. 14.2). Special attention should be paid to the foods (◻ Table 14.2), which can cause discomfort, for example, due to insufficient chewing, solid or fibrous structures or unintentional swallowing. By recording them in a diet and complaints diary, patients can be sensitised to specific intolerances and sensible avoidance strategies can be discussed in the consultation.

14.2 Long-Term Nutrition After Bariatric Surgery

H. Berger

Long-term nutrition after bariatric surgery is the form of nutrition that is permanently recommended after the initial postoperative diet regimen. Just like in the three stages explained above, it is intended to prevent the development of malnutrition and nutrition-related complaints. The rules of eating behaviour (▶ Sect. 14.1) have to be observed constantly. So far, only a few authors have dealt with long-term nutrition after bariatric surgery. Moizé et al. (2010) have developed a nutrition pyramid (◻ Fig. 14.1) for gastric bypass patients based on a diet low in fat and rich in protein and fibre. The use of this pyramid as nutritional advice for patients undergoing other bariatric procedures, such as a sleeve gastrectomy, should be investigated in future studies.

Dietary complications can occur both during the initial postoperative diet regimen and—to a lesser extent—during long-term nutrition at a later stage. Complications are, for example

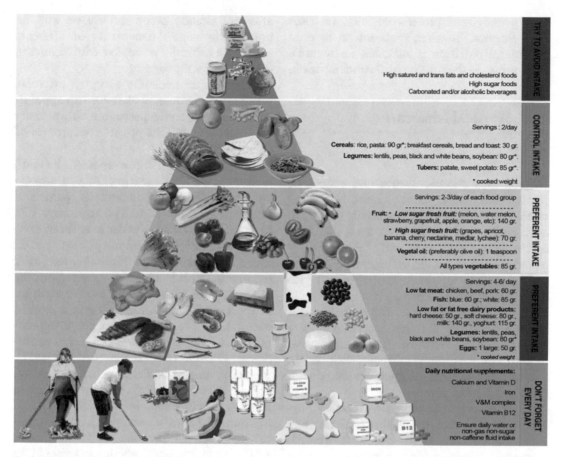

Fig. 14.1 Food pyramid for patients undergoing gastric bypass surgery. (Mod. according to Moizé et al. 2010)

- Dumping syndrome,
- Nausea and vomiting,
- Meteorism,
- Diarrhea,
- Constipation,
- Food intolerances,
- Dehydration.

Recurring complaints require further diagnostics and therapeutic measures, in which renewed nutritional advice in particular plays a decisive role.

14.3 Supplementation

H. Berger

In obese patients, a lack of vitamins or minerals may already exist before bariatric interventions due to unbalanced nutrition (Saltzmann and Karl 2013). Possible deficiency symptoms should be diagnosed and compensated for in advance of bariatric surgery. Depending on the surgical procedure, anatomical changes of the digestive tract may occur, resulting in different degrees of malabsorptive effects.

In restrictive procedures, such as sleeve gastrectomy, deficiency symptoms occur less frequently after surgery than in malabsorptive procedures, such as gastric bypass surgery and biliopancreatic diversion (Handzlik-Orlik et al. 2014). In addition, low food intake, intolerances and developing aversions to certain foods or groups of foods can lead to the development of nutrient deficiencies. The deficiency of macro- and micronutrients can persist in bariatric patients and thus make lifelong supplementation necessary (see also ▶ Sect. 14.5.2). To avoid a protein deficiency, the intake of 60–120 g of protein per day is recommended. If possible, this should be ensured by a protein-rich diet. In cases of deficiency, however, oral, enteral or even parenteral nutrition is indicated for therapy, depending on the severity of the malnutrition.

14.4 Surgical Aftercare

J. Ordemann

Obesity is a chronic disease and cannot be treated curatively. Thus, surgically treated obesity patients remain chronically (obese) ill and require lifelong therapy, even if they have lost weight significantly and their secondary diseases have improved. Aftercare should not only focus on weight development but also on changes in secondary diseases, nutritional deficiencies, complications and quality of life.

Studies show that patients who receive professional aftercare are significantly better able to lose weight and maintain their weight loss in the long term than patients who do not receive this aftercare.

It is crucial that competent obesity physicians coordinate this follow-up care and refer patients to other specialists (plastic surgeons, cardiologists, pulmonologists) if necessary. Patients who signal avoidance of aftercare already preoperatively or who do not acknowledge the necessity of aftercare should be critically evaluated with regard to the indication for surgery.

There is no generally excepted aftercare scheme. The frequency of follow-up appointments depends on the procedure, the intensity of weight loss and the possible occurrence of complications.

The first surgical follow-up is on the tenth postoperative day. During this follow-up visit, wound healing, presence of pain, and problems with the initial postoperative diet regimen are assessed in order to rule out early postoperative complications. Since weight loss is most pronounced in the first year after the operation, it is advisable to carry out the aftercare at regular intervals every 3 months. In the second year, follow-up every 6 months is sufficient. From the third year postoperatively, annual follow-up is supposed to be sufficient (◘ Table 14.3). If, however, internal or psychosomatic complications or complaints arise, the aftercare should be carried out more closely again (▶ Sects. 14.5 and 14.6).

Surgical follow-up should assess the clinical condition of the patient. In particular, BMI and excess body weight loss should be carefully recorded. It is important to con-

14

◘ **Table 14.3**   Aftercare scheme

	10 days postop.	Week 4	Month 3	Month 6	Month 9	Month 12	Month 18	Month 24	Month 36	Month 48	Yearly
Surgeon, nutritionist	X	x	x	x	x	x	x	x	x	x	x
Internist, endocrinologist		x		x		x		x		x	x
Psychologist			x[1]			x[1]			x[1]		x[1]

x[1] if necessary

tinuously document these data in order to be able to react early on to a renewed increase in weight. The core task of surgical aftercare is to identify complications. Depending on the surgical procedure (gastric banding, sleeve gastrectomy or gastric bypass), the symptoms vary and require adequate diagnostics and therapy (► Sect. 14.7).

> **Practical Tip**
>
> All medical information should be carefully recorded as part of the follow-up care and inserted into a database of obesity surgery quality assurance.

14.5 Internal Aftercare

U. Elbelt

The task of internal aftercare is the adjustment of the pre-existing medication during postoperative weight reduction, the early identification of nutrition-related deficiencies, the appropriate treatment of obesity-related pre-existing diseases as well as the treatment of additional cardiovascular risk factors, which mostly occur in the context of a metabolic syndrome. Following the postoperative phase of "effortless" weight reduction, further care is aimed at preventing renewed weight gain. At each presentation, the patient's current complaints, eating habits, weight development, changes in existing comorbidities and current life circumstances should be assessed. In addition, weight measurement and a careful physical examination are required. Aftercare has to be provided throughout the patient's postoperative life.

14.5.1 Follow-Up in the Early Postoperative Phase

The initial postoperative dietary regimen is described in detail in ► Sect. 14.1. In the early postoperative phase, the internal follow-up focuses on complaints with food intake and the adjustment of the pre-existing medication.

The medical history should specifically ask about pain associated with food intake and the frequency of vomiting. Should *vomiting* occur repeatedly, a (renewed) detailed nutritional consultation and, if necessary, a psychosomatic presentation is necessary. Surgical complications (► Sect. 14.7) have to be ruled out beforehand. Immediately before surgery, *oral antidiabetics* (especially metformin and insulinotropic substances with the potential to cause hypoglycaemia) should be discontinued if type 2 diabetes mellitus is present. In the case of pre-existing *insulin therapy*, the administration of basal insulin should be at least halved postoperatively; prandial insulin administration should first be paused. In order to be able to react appropriately to the early drop in insulin requirements (within the first postoperative week), a 4-point daily blood glucose profile should be carried out regularly during the inpatient stay. Postoperatively elevated blood glucose levels should be compensated for by short-acting insulin in a reduced dose.

> **Practical Tip**
>
> These recommendations must not be applied to patients with diabetes mellitus type 1. In these patients, too, there is usually a drastic reduction in insulin requirements. Changes in basal insulin coverage, modification of daytime dependent insulin/carbohydrate-ratios and reduction of the insulin correction factor should be discussed in detail with the patient and the treating diabetologist prior to surgery.

Furthermore, in this phase, the therapy with *diuretics* has to be adjusted to avoid dehydration and hypokalemia. An antihypertensive medication should also be reduced, if necessary.

14.5.2 Aftercare During the Weight Loss Phase ('Honeymoon Phase')

The "honeymoon phase"covers the first 18 (up to max. 24) months postoperatively. Its end is marked by renewed weight gain or no further weight loss.

The weight loss is most pronounced in the first 6 postoperative months. In this phase, the reduction of *antihypertensive therapy* and also a possible pre-existing *therapy with thyroid hormones* is of particular importance. During this time, a drug therapy to *prevent gallstone formation* with ursodeoxycholic acid in a dosage of at least 500 mg/day for a period of 6 months should be administered. Whether a drug prophylaxis for prevention of gout attacks is necessary is still a matter of debate. In our centre, this is only done in a targeted manner.

During this phase, the psychosomatic symptom burden is generally reduced and the psychosocial level of function improves. As a result, the psychosomatic aftercare offer is no longer perceived necessary by most patients, so that potential psychological problems have to be assessed as part of internal aftercare. Especially for women who have undergone surgery, the temporary *increased hair loss* that occurs in the third month after the operation is very stressful. This usually lasts for 3–6 months. Treatment with biotin and consistent iron supplementation are recommended. The topical constant application of hair tonic containing minoxidil (and estradiol) is effective after a latency period. Being cold is also often reported to be very unpleasant. With continued weight loss, the *burden of skin sagging* increases. These should be inspected in order to prevent inflammatory skin changes and to initiate therapy at an early stage. Careful documentation is particularly important for justifying the necessity of plastic surgery that is planned in the further course of weight loss. However, these operations should generally only be performed after weight reduction has been completed in a phase of weight stability (usually not until the 18th postoperative month). Due to the change in appearance and lifestyle, partnership conflicts can often occur in this phase.

Some patients are burdened by the occurrence of *diarrhoea* and associated faecal incontinence. Since this is often not reported out of shame, it should be specifically asked for. Differential diagnoses include gastroin-

testinal infections (which are favoured by the postoperative lack of an acid barrier in the stomach), bacterial colonisation of the small intestine and relative lactose intolerance. It is helpful to carry out targeted medical investigations.

With regard to the use of *medication*, altered *absorption* should be considered, especially after gastric bypass surgery. Especially the therapy with oral anticoagulants and anticonvulsants should be closely monitored. Women have to be informed of the reduced effectiveness of oral contraceptives. Alternative contraceptive methods should therefore be used for safe contraception. Overall, liquid pharmaceutical preparations appear to be more favourable with regard to absorption. In this context, the postoperative higher *alcohol sensitivity* due to faster absorption should also be pointed out. The consumption of alcohol should be assessed and discussed at every follow-up visit.

Especially after gastric bypass surgery, the avoidance of macro- and micronutrient *deficiencies* is of central importance in internal aftercare. While to our experience a protein deficiency tends to be a minor problem, special attention should be paid to the avoidance of *hypovitaminosis D_3* with subsequent development of secondary hyperparathyroidism, iron deficiency anaemia and *hypovitaminosis B_{12}*.

To avoid deficiencies, consistent postoperative supplementation and regular laboratory testing should be carried out for an early detection. The symptoms of a micronutrient deficiency can be very diverse. For this reason, a (previously overlooked) deficiency should always be considered for differential diagnosis in the case of reported complaints or conspicuous clinical findings.

Supplementation should include multivitamin administration, additional intake of calcium, vitamin D_3 and iron, and parenteral administration of vitamin B_{12}.

Hypovitaminosis D_3 is often present preoperatively and should be compensated for prior to the operation. Postoperatively, the need for supplementation is increased and after gastric bypass surgery it may often be necessary to take up to 5000 IU of vitamin D_3 daily. To avoid secondary hyperparathyroidism, in addition to supplementation of vitamin D_3, sufficient calcium intake must be ensured. The intake of calcium citrate is preferred to calcium carbonate.

In particular, menstruating women have a high risk of developing *iron deficiency anaemia* postoperatively. In addition to the postoperative reduced production of gastric acid, proton pump inhibitors are frequently taken. If sleeve gastrectomy is performed, anaemia results from a reduced ferrous iron leading to decreased absorption in the duodenum and proximal jejunum. The oral administration of iron can cause constipation. Due to the undesirable side effects, intravenous administration should only be used in cases of iron deficiency that are refractory to therapy. Before this, however, gastrointestinal blood loss should be excluded by appropriate diagnostics (which is more difficult in gastric bypass surgery).

On the one hand, the surgically induced reduction of the stomach volume by sleeve gastrectomy leads to a lack of intrinsic factor, on the other hand, after gastric bypass surgery, the duodenal formation of vitamin B_{12} intrinsic factor complex with uptake in the terminal ileum is diminished, so that vitamin B_{12} must be administered parenterally. The postoperative need for vitamin B_{12} is highly variable. In most cases, the administration of 1000 µg of vitamin B_{12} at three-month intervals intramuscularly or injected deeply subcutaneously is sufficient. The consequences of *hypovitaminosis B_{12}* can be megaloblastic anaemia, peripheral polyneuropathy (PNP) or funicular myelosis.

A *folic acid deficiency* can also lead to anaemia and/or neurological symptoms. Usually, 300–400 µg daily are supplied in the form of a multivitamin preparation. Particularly in women who wish to have children after bariatric surgery, adequate folic acid substitution should be ensured, since a folic acid deficiency can promote the development of neural tube defects.

In the case of recurrent vomiting, thiamine deficiency (*hypovitaminosis B_1*) should be excluded, which may result from a combination of reduced intake, vomiting and malabsorption, especially after gastric bypass surgery. The risk of Wernicke-Korsakow syndrome should be considered. Initially, at least 100–250 mg of thiamine should be administered intravenously daily and oral therapy should only be given once the symptoms have improved.

A detailed overview of the recommended supplementation is given in ◻ Table 14.4.

◻ **Table 14.4** Supplementation recommendations after bariatric surgery[a]

Micronutrient	Dose		
	Gastric band	**Sleeve gastrectomy**	**Gastric bypass**
Calcium(citrate)	1200–1500 mg/day	1200–1500 mg/day	1200–1500 mg/day
Vitamin D_3	1000–2000 IU/day	2000–3000 IU/day	2000–3000 IU/day
Vitamin B_{12}		1000 µg every 3 months i. m.	1000 µg every 3 months i. m.
Multivitamin preparation with minerals and trace elements	1×/day	1×/day	1–2×/day
Iron (especially for menstruating women)			100 mg/day for deficiency

[a]Individual adaptation of the supplementation recommendations according to laboratory testing and clinical complaints is necessary

14.5.3 Aftercare in the Phase of Weight Stagnation or Weight Regain

Approximately 12–18 months postoperatively the weight nadir is reached and in most cases, there is renewed weight gain. In this phase, the identification of causes is of decisive importance. More often than not, a feeling of inadequate satiety has returned, meal portions are getting larger and eating habits are approaching those that existed before the operation. The weight gain leads to shame and fear. A renewed close accompanying nutritional consultation can be very helpful. Postoperative suicides occur especially in the third postoperative year. Especially in this vulnerable phase of aftercare, the intervals between follow-up visits are extended in many centres. For this reason, a regular follow-up should take place especially in the phase of beginning weight gain. These frequently occurring difficulties illustrate the importance of psychosomatic aftercare, which is also useful in the case of initial postoperative well-being. If this has not taken place, it is now reasonable to initiate renewed psychosomatic support as part of the internal presentation.

14.5.4 Recommended Aftercare Intervals

So far there is no binding recommendation on the follow-up intervals. Usually, the aftercare is carried out in the following intervals:
- Gastric banding: every 3 months in the first postoperative year, then annually
- Gastric bypass: every 3 months in the first postoperative year, every 6 months in the second postoperative year, then at least annually.

For the above-mentioned reasons, after all bariatric surgeries, the first post-operative care in our centre is 4–6 weeks postoperatively, then 3, 6, 9 and 12 months post-operatively. In the second post-operative year, patients come every 6 months, and then usually every year. However, in the third post-operative year, follow-up care is also often arranged every 6 months. Within the framework of structured aftercare, our patients do not always have to present themselves at all the clinics involved in the aftercare. However, there is close coordination between the individual disciplines.

14.5.5 Recommended Laboratory Diagnostics

There is also no consensus to date regarding the necessary laboratory testing. The following parameters should be determined in the controls:
- Routine: blood count, total protein, albumin, transaminases, cholestasis parameters, electrolytes, calcium, renal retention parameters, uric acid, vitamin B_{12}, folic acid, ferritin, vitamin D_3, PTH, INR after malabsorptive procedures;
- Co-morbidity related: blood glucose, HbA_{1c}, total cholesterol, LDL cholesterol, HDL cholesterol, triglycerides, TSH;
- Symptom-based: zinc, thiamine, vitamin A.

> **Practical Tip**
>
> The extent of micronutrient deficiencies increases from gastric banding, sleeve gastrectomy, gastric bypass to (only rarely performed) biliopancreatic diversion. This has to be taken into account for an adequate supplementation, planning of follow-up intervals and the frequency of laboratory testing.

14.6 Psychosomatic Aftercare

T. Hofmann

The necessity of postoperative psychosomatic aftercare is derived from the high psychological stress of the treated patient group. Even though serious psychosocial complications are rare, special attention should be paid to the development of addictions and suicidal thoughts. Further aspects of aftercare include eating behaviour, mood, and the assessment of quality of life and changes in social roles.

According to the current S3 guideline on obesity surgery, patients after bariatric surgery require regular follow-up care by a physician experienced in obesity therapy as well as competent nutritional advice. Psychosomatic aftercare can therefore be recommended in cases of pre-operative mental disorders or post-operative loss of control eating and further mental disorders after bariatric surgery. It should be added that the treatment of manifest mental disorders is not only recommended but is always indicated, even independently of any somatic illnesses that may be present. This is even more true after bariatric surgery, which has to be regarded as a drastic life event with considerable physical changes.

While the suspicion of a depression, an anxiety disorder or the (re)appearance of loss of control over food intake should in any case lead to a psychosomatic presentation, the question of whether a regular psychosomatic evaluation after bariatric surgery should also be carried out in patients with preoperative mental well-being, is less clear.

From a more fundamental point of view, a cursory psychosocial evaluation should be part of every—somatic—medical treatment. In this regard, the interdisciplinary treatment approach for obese patients is already considerably more advanced compared to other fields of somatic medicine. The need for psychosomatic co-care of bariatric patients also arises from the enormously high rate of concomitant mental disorders in this group (▶ Sect. 1.5), which are also associated with a poorer postoperative outcome.

It is unclear, however, to what extent and how often psychosomatic evaluations should take place. In the sense of optimal care, more or less short examinations should also be aimed for within the framework of established surgical and internal aftercare, i.e., usually 6 weeks, 3 months, 6 months and 12 months after surgery and then at annual intervals. Certainly, such postoperative screening for psychosocial problems does not necessarily have to be carried out by a specialist in psychosomatic medicine. It would be conceivable that not only the psychosomatic, but

also the entire postoperative follow-up care is carried out by doctors experienced in the care of obese patients and in basic psychosomatic care. This form of care would have the advantage that the aftercare could be carried out by one person in an integrated manner. In view of the increasing number of bariatric operations, which will certainly continue to rise, and thus also the cumulative enormously increased need for aftercare, such models would be desirable anyway, at least for basic care. This basic care could be supported by the use of psychometric questionnaires, which are well validated and can be used with minimal time required. To date additive forms of specialised surgical, internal as well as psychosomatic care carried out to different times and at different places are more common. It would be desirable for integrated postoperative care to be provided in teams at one place.

In psychosomatic aftercare, the current eating habits should be questioned regularly. In particular, it is important to address the meal-related daytime structure, possible nighttime eating (up to night-eating syndrome) and the occurrence of hunger pangs (up to binge-eating disorder). In addition, unfavourable eating behaviour has to be addressed. This includes, for example, "grazing", in which unstructured eating is spread throughout the day, or "sweet eating", in which large quantities of sweet foods, sweets and often especially sweetened drinks (such as soft drinks) are consumed. The consumption of sweetened drinks or other liquid foods can play a role, especially after bariatric surgery, as this is a way of circumventing the restrictive mechanism of bariatric surgery. The eating behaviour displayed after bariatric surgery seems to be a stronger predictor of achievable weight loss compared to the preoperatively assessed eating behaviour.

All forms of vomiting have to be assessed. While vomiting is a phenomenon that can be observed immediately after surgery in adaptation to the changed anatomical conditions, a possible chronification should be recognized and addressed early. Especially, attention should be paid to self-induced vomiting, which may occur as an attempt to accelerate weight loss; however, self-induced vomiting can also be an expression of a shifting or newly occurring eating disorder.

Attention should also be paid to the mood of the patients. Even if the majority of patients tends to be in an almost euphoric mood, especially in the first few months of the often rapid weight loss, individual patients may experience mood swings that may even lead to manifest depression or anxiety disorders, for example, as a reaction to the lack of possibilities to compensate for emotional states through food intake or—less frequently—due to massive changes in body image. The latter sometimes also plays a role with regard to changes in social relationships and here especially in partnerships. These changes are by no means always perceived as positive. The pronounced, not only physical change of a partner may be associated with unfavourable changes in a couple's relationship.

In addition to depressive illnesses and uncontrolled eating habits, the regain of body weight seems to be associated with emotionally unstable and impulsive personality traits, abuse of alcohol and other drugs, but also less use of (somatic) aftercare appointments. In addition to adherence to aftercare, the implementation of recommendations on physical activity and nutrition patterns also plays an important role, which is largely dependent on psychological, and especially social factors. Adherence to aftercare appointments seems to decrease postoperatively if adherence was limited already preoperatively.

Further important aspects in psychosomatic aftercare are the first occurrence or recurrence of addictions, especially alcohol abuse, or life-weary thoughts, including manifest suicidal tendencies. Empirical data suggest an increased risk for these conditions in comparison to non-operated patients. As patients often conceal these conditions, active and regular enquiries questioning is recommended. In contrast, depression usually improves postoperatively.

In this context it is important to note that the main proportion of suicides seems to be between 1 and 4 years after surgery. In this time period patients frequently experience weight regain and the length of post-operative care intervals usually increase. It may become critical if weight regain and decreasing medical care, perceived by most patients as a change for the worse, meet with increasing hopelessness, a negative body experience or interpersonal problems. Patients might experience that the operative change in body weight has not led to the hoped-for changes in regard to overall satisfaction and that psychological instabilities have persisted. In addition to unfulfilled expectations regarding the success of the operative measure, changes in previously stable personal relationships and partnerships, including sexual life, should not be underestimated.

> **Topics of Psychosomatic Postoperative Aftercare**
> - Assessment of mood and emotions (especially depressive and anxiety symptoms)
> - Life-weary thoughts and suicidal tendencies
> - Eating behaviour (loss of control, eating at night, sweet eating, grazing, vomiting)
> - Development of substance abuse and addictions (especially alcohol, but also other substance-bound and behavioural addictions)
> - Assessment of mental and physical quality of life and social role function

Continued low-threshold access to psychosomatic services is particularly recommended because long-term improvement of mental well-being cannot be assumed regularly. In a follow-up study up to 9 years after restrictive bariatric surgery, depressive symptoms and especially anxiety symptoms increased again in patients who had undergone surgery after initial improvement. These deteriorations were not associated with changes in BMI and were not observed in patients receiving conservative therapy. The initial improvements of various aspects of health-related quality of life are also shown to decline over the long term in several studies. These findings illustrate the psychosocial care needs of this highly burdened patient group.

Structured aftercare programmes, primarily behavioural and eating behaviour-oriented, can support postoperative success in terms of more pronounced weight loss. While most of the heterogeneous aftercare programs investigated so far started directly postoperatively, the phase of weight stagnation or regaining weight about 18 months after surgery could be a suitable target for postoperative interventions. Due to the very high prevalence of mental disorders, the integration of differentiated psychosocial interventions into the aftercare programmes would be desirable. In addition, guided or self-organised self-help groups can be supportive.

14.7 Surgical Complications

C. Menenakos and J. Ordemann

With the rapid development of obesity surgery, the knowledge of possible complications of the corresponding surgery procedures has also increased.

The complication rate depends on the surgical procedure performed. Depending on the time of occurrence, complications are divided into:

- early complications, including postoperative anastomotic leak or staple suture insufficiency, iatrogenic perforation, postoperative bleeding, intestinal obstruction, and
- later complications, including slippage of the gastric band, stenoses, reflux, chole(cysto)lithiasis and dumping syndromes.

Knowledge of the anatomical changes caused by the respective bariatric surgical procedures is essential for understanding and targeted treatment of possible complications.

14.7.1 Early Surgical Complications

Early complications are characterized by their occurrence within the first days after surgery. Timely diagnosis of these complications is crucial, as delayed treatment can have life-threatening consequences. The most important early postoperative complications include leakage (anastomosis or suture failure), bleeding and obstruction.

Postoperative Leak

The symptoms of patients with early postoperative leaks can be manifold. Acute pain, tachycardia, tachypnoea and fever are indicative; some of these symptoms may also be absent. If a drain was placed intraoperatively, turbid secretion can be a direct indication of a leak.

In case of a high-grade suspicion of anastomotic leak or staple suture insufficiency, direct surgical revision is recommended. The necessary diagnostics has to be performed quickly and targeted. Conventional X-ray diagnostics is playing an increasingly subordinate role. Computed tomography (CT) of the abdomen with an oral water-soluble contrast medium is the diagnostic procedure of choice for imaging postoperative leaks (❏ Fig. 14.2).

As soon as the diagnosis of a leak is confirmed, a calculated antibiotic therapy must be administered immediately. In addition, an antifungal therapy is recommended for leaks in the area of the stomach or the gastroesophageal junction.

The earlier a postoperative leak occurs and is diagnosed, the more promising is secondary surgical oversewing of the insufficiency. This is followed by lavage of the surgical area and,

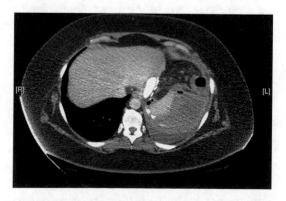

❏ **Fig. 14.2** Contrast agent computed tomography of the upper abdomen: Status after sleeve gastrectomy, proximal leakage with abscess formation

as an essential aspect of revision surgery, the placement of drains in the area of the insufficiency. Surgical oversewing of the leak is only recommended if it can be performed within 3 days of the occurrence of the insufficiency. Later oversewing is usually unsuccessful due to the massive inflammatory reaction in the area of the insufficiency which has occurred in the meantime. The removal of an abscess caused by the leak and the insertion of drains are necessary in any case. This can be done conservatively with CT support.

Deviating from the recommendations mentioned above, proven insufficiency of a small intestine anastomosis due to leak of bile has to be surgically revised in any case.

In the case of proven insufficiency, fasting of the patient is required. Nutrition should initially be parenteral. Some authors recommend the immediate insertion of a gastric tube to ensure drain of gastric secretion. If a significantly delayed start of postoperative oral diet regimen is to be expected, enteral feeding should be ensured by placing a feeding tube. This should already be considered during the revision procedure.

Postoperative Bleeding

Bleeding is a dramatic complication of bariatric surgery that must be diagnosed and treated immediately. Classic signs of post-operative bleeding are tachycardia, malaise and as the case may be impairment of circulation. If there is simultaneous hematemesis or bloody secretion via drains, further diagnostics and therapy have to be initiated immediately. More rarely, hematochezia may occur, which indicates a massive intraluminal hemorrhage.

Basically, bleeding can occur intraluminally or intra-abdominally. The intraluminal bleeding originates from staple sutures and can often be diagnosed endoscopically and treated simultaneously. Intra-abdominal bleeding can originate from various bleeding sites, such as splenic injuries, staple suture line, omentum injuries, the Aa./Vv. gastricae breves and trocar incision sites. If these bleedings do not stop, the surgical revision has be to initiated immediately.

Therapeutic intervention includes measures to stabilize the circulation, such as infusion therapy and, if necessary, transfusions, as well as the discontinuation of anticoagulants and fasting. Careful clinical monitoring is indicated.

If there are indications of intraluminal bleeding in the stomach pouch or the gastric sleeve, an endoscopy of the upper gastrointestinal tract has to be performed. If a safe hemostasis cannot be achieved by endoscopic intervention, an emergency revision surgery is necessary.

In the case of suspected intra-abdominal bleeding in (still) circulatory stable patients, computer tomographic diagnostics is recommended first for localizing bleeding sites and also hematomas.

If there are clear indications of intra-abdominal bleeding in patients with circulatory instability, immediate surgical revision in the form of a relaparoscopy is recommended for diagnostics, localization of bleeding, hemostasis and hematoma removal. If the bleeding cannot be stopped laparoscopically, surgery has to be converted to a laparotomy at an early stage.

Postoperative Obstruction

Stenoses or obstructions after bariatric surgery are rare, but they represent an extremely dangerous complication and must be treated immediately. After gastric bypass operations (RYGB), obstructive complications are significantly more frequent than after sleeve gastrectomy.

Depending on the location of the obstruction, the condition of the patients differs significantly. Besides recurrent vomiting and malaise, patients may also show clear signs of an ileus with shock symptoms.

Obstruction or stenosis can occur in the area of the pouch anastomosis, but also in the area of the entero-entero-anastomosis. These stenoses can be caused by an inaccurate anastomosis technique as well as by kinking of intestinal loops and oedematous swelling of the anastomosis. In addition, internal hernias or bridles play an important role in the genesis of obstructions.

Obstructions lead to an accumulation of fluid, chyme, gastric and bile secretions. The accumulation of these fluids leads secondarily to a dilatation of the upstream sections of the gastrointestinal tract. A stenosis in the area of the gastrojejunostomy leads directly to an inability of fluid intake. Regurgitation occurs. Immediate diagnosis with X-ray contrast imaging and gastroscopy is indicated. Stenoses in the area of jejuno-jejunostomy induce an accumulation of intestinal secretions into the alimentary and/or biliopancreatic loop. This leads to dilatation of the affected loop or the remaining stomach. This is an acute, life-threatening clinical picture. Immediate sonographic and radiological diagnostics with subsequent laparoscopic revision is indicated.

In addition, stenosis or obstruction can be caused by internal hernias, which make a direct surgical revision necessary. Hernias typical for gastric bypass surgery in the Petersen's space or in the area of entero-entero-anastomosis are described below.

Early Complications After Gastric Band Implantation

Injury to the stomach wall during implantation of a gastric band (LAGB) is extremely rare. However, if an injury to the dorsal stomach wall or the oesophagus occurs intraoperatively, the mortality rate is high. In most cases, these injuries occur when the stomach is tunnelled dorsally. In case of clinical suspicion, computer tomography is necessary. The immediate surgical revision with removal of the gastric band and oversewing the leak is necessary.

Bleeding after LAGB is also very rare. Bleedings are mostly caused by injuries of the small curvature and retrogastric tunnel area. Surgical visualization of the source of bleeding and hemostasis are often difficult. If it is not possible to visualize the bleeding, it may be necessary to inspect the posterior wall of the stomach by sealing and cutting through the Aa./Vv. gastric breves.

There are various forms of inaccurate implantation of a gastric band. For example, the gastric band may be placed too far proximally, around the oesophagus, or too far distally around the stomach. If the band is inaccurately placed around the esophagus, there is no gastric pouch. Patients complain

of dysphagia, and secondary oesophageal dilatation may occur. A too low position leads to a higher pouch volume and consequently to less weight loss.

Surgical repositioning of the gastric band is indicated in these cases. The gastric band should be applied using the pars flaccida technique to create a small gastric pouch. If necessary, a tube with a calibration balloon can be inserted into the stomach. To avoid further slippage, it is recommended to fix the band with a gastric plication (▶ Chap. 8).

Early Complications After a Sleeve Gastrectomy

The rate of staple suture insufficiencies after sleeve gastrectomy (LSG) is reported in the literature to be 0.3–7.8%. Approximately 75% of staple suture insufficiencies after LSG affect the gastroesophageal junction.

Several studies have investigated the influence of staple suture reinforcement or oversewing of the staple suture on insufficiency rate. Despite contradictory results in the single studies, Gagner and Buchwald (2014) were able to show a slight advantage for the reinforcement of the staple line in a systematic review (88 studies with 8920 patients). In a meta-analysis by Parikh et al. (2013) it was found that the staple suture insufficiency rate was reduced when using a calibration tube of >40 F. In this work, the use of staple line reinforcement showed no effect on the suture insufficiency rate. A final evaluation with valid treatment recommendations can therefore not be made at present.

As stated above, early operative revision is indicated. If safe surgical closure by oversewing the suture insufficiency is not promising or not possible, various conservative treatment options are available. Best established are the insertion of a covered stent, the endoscopic application of "over the scope clips" (OTSC), the endoscopic introduction of a sponge system or the internal drainage using a pigtail catheter. The indication for the use of these different procedures depends on the size of the leak, the time of diagnosis and the endoscopic expertise. Final recommendations for the respective procedures cannot be given yet.

The frequency of postoperative bleeding after LSG is given in the literature as 1–6%. The use of staple line reinforcement seems to reduce the postoperative bleeding rate.

> **Practical Tip**
>
> If staple line hemorrhage is detected, a staple suture insufficiency may be present at the same time. The latter has to be excluded.

Postoperative stenoses after LSG have become very rare due to the consistent use of calibration tubes. Often these stenoses were found in the area of the incisura angularis. The possible formation of a secondary suture insufficiency above the constriction is problematic. Clinically, nausea and repeated vomiting indicate the presence of a stenosis. For diagnostics, a conventional X-ray of the stomach with oral administration of a water-soluble contrast medium and gastroscopy are indicated. In the case of stenosis, the treatment of choice is a temporary endoscopic stent implantation (usually for a period of 4 weeks). In the case of early postoperative stenosis, balloon dilatation is not an alternative treatment because of the considerable risk of rupture of the staple line.

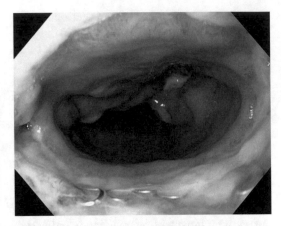

◘ **Fig. 14.3**   Gastroscopy: anastomotic leak in the area of gastrojejunostomy after gastric bypass surgery

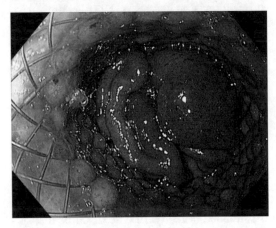

◘ **Fig. 14.4**   Gastroscopy: stent implantation in case of an anastomotic leak

Early Complications After Gastric Bypass

The incidence of anastomotic leak or suture insufficiency after RYGB is up to 5% and is a decisive factor for postoperative mortality in this patient group. The gastrojejunal pouch anastomosis is the most frequently affected (◘ Fig. 14.3). The principles described above apply for diagnostics and treatment (see above, postoperative leak).

In addition to the surgical revision of early detected leaks in the area of gastrojejunal anastomosis after RYGB, alternative conservative therapeutic strategies are increasingly applied. These include the endoscopic insertion of covered stents and the use of OTSC for endoscopic closure of the leak. The insertion of covered stents is used to temporarily cover the leak (◘ Fig. 14.4).

It should be considered that stents can cause considerable discomfort for some patients (pain, reflux, nausea). Furthermore, the risk of a possible migration of stents must be taken into account. Stent removal is usually carried out after 4 weeks. When using OTSCs, it should be noted that the abscess cavities formed by the insufficiency have to be drained.

In contrast, distal leaks of the small intestine anastomosis have to be surgically revised in any case. If the inflammation of the peritoneum is still locally limited, an oversewing is usually sufficient in case of small anastomotic leaks. In advanced peritonitis or greater anastomotic leaks, a new small bowel anastomosis is indicated. In septic patients with 4-quadrant peritonitis a stoma formation should be considered.

14

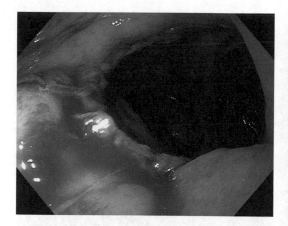

◘ Fig. 14.5 Gastroscopy: intraluminal bleeding in the area of the anastomosis after gastric bypass surgery

Significant postoperative bleeding requiring transfusion occurs in approximately 1–4% of patients after RYGB. Here too, a distinction must be made between intraluminal and intra-abdominal bleeding (◘ Fig. 14.5). Often, post-operative bleeding after RYGB can be well controlled by conservative measures. However, in up to 25% of cases of early postoperative bleeding, surgical revision is necessary. There are also indications in the literature that reinforcing the staple line could reduce the post-operative bleeding rate.

A stenosis in the area of the pouch anastomosis is often the result of an incorrect surgical technique. Postoperative stenoses after circular staple suture technique are less frequent than after linear staple anastomosis or manual suturing. Patients with a stenosis in the area of the gastric pouch anastomosis can hardly take in any fluids following the operation. Massive vomiting is generally not possible. If an anastomotic stenosis is suspected, immediate diagnostics by means of X-ray contrast passage and gastroscopy is necessary (◘ Figs. 14.6 and 14.7). In case of complete obstruction, a new anastomosis is indicated. If a partial stenosis is present, it is possible to monitor the patient and wait for some time. Early endoscopic dilatation is not recommended due to the risk of rupture of the staple line. In case of additional edema, patients often experience improvement of the symptoms within a few days after the operation due to a reduction in swelling. In older

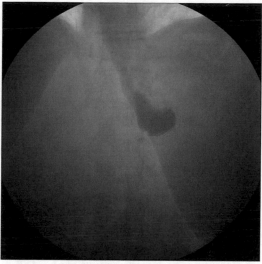

◘ Fig. 14.6 X-ray: gastric pouch after gastric bypass surgery. Complete stop of the contrast medium due to stenosis

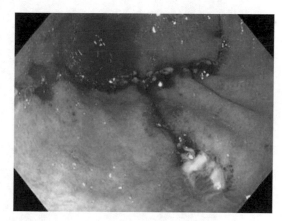

◘ Fig. 14.7 Gastroscopy: complete obstruction of the gastrojejunostomy after gastric bypass surgery

stenoses, dilatation is the therapy of choice (▶ Sect. 14.7.2).

Stenoses in the area of distal small bowel anastomosis can clinically appear much more dramatic. An accumulation in the alimentary loop quickly leads to malaise, vomiting of undigested food, but also to colic and tachycardia. In this case, CT diagnostics are confirmative and surgical correction is necessary.

An accumulation in the biliopancreatic loop can lead to a life-threatening situation in a short time. Radiologically, dilated loops of the small intestine and the dilated stomach (stomach distension) are a clear sign of an obstruction. At the same time, there is an increase in liver enzymes, cholestatic parameters, lipase and inflammation markers. Immediate laparoscopic therapy is indicated. The stomach should be decompressed independently of stenosis resolution of the small intestine anastomosis, with the aim to avoid a staple line rupture of the remaining stomach. Decompression can be achieved intraoperatively by means of a gastrostomy, which is closed again after decompression.

Obstructions due to hernias can be manifold. In gastric bypass surgery explicit reference is made to the hernias in the area of the Petersen's space. In addition, abdominal wall hernia at the site of trocar incisions can lead to classical obstruction symptoms as well as vital endangerment of patients. This topic will be discussed further in the next section.

14.7.2 Late Surgical Complications

Late surgical complications become manifest weeks to years after the operation. Late surgical complications after bariatric surgery include slippage of the gastric band, stenoses after LSG and RYGB, reflux, chole(cysto)lithiasis and dumping syndromes. Since the occurrence of these complications depends especially on the type of bariatric surgery, late surgical complications are discussed separately for each surgical procedure.

Late Complications After Gastric Band Implantation

The LAGB has a very low rate of early postoperative mortality and morbidity. However, this procedure can lead to late surgical complications, so that the longer-term re-operation rate for LAGB is reported to be 10–20%. The main complication is the so-called gastric band slippage, which occurs in up to 6% of patients after LAGB. An anterior and a posterior form of slippage can be distinguished. An anterior slippage occurs significantly more frequently. Usual complaints of the patients are obstructive symptoms like dysphagia and belching, epigastric pain and reflux symptoms.

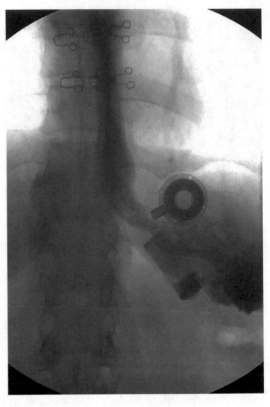

Fig. 14.8 X-ray image of the stomach: slippage after gastric banding

Stomach passage with oral contrast medium is the radiological method of choice for the diagnosis of slippage. The gastric band shows up rather in a horizontal position. In addition, a dilated pouch proximal to the gastric band and a decelerated passage of the contrast medium may be detected (**Fig. 14.8**).

In contrast to slippage, the radiological signs of pouch dilatation without slippage of the gastric band are a symmetrical enlargement of the pouch with inconspicuous position of the gastric band. In case of pouch dilatation, patients have chronic, mild symptoms such as reflux symptoms, reduced feeling of fullness and possibly intermittent pain in the left upper abdomen, but without the symptoms of acute obstruction mentioned above.

The therapy of choice is removal of liquid from the port system. Often this already leads to an improvement of the symptoms.

14

Since gastric band slippage leads to symptomatic exsiccosis of the patients, rehydration should be ensured immediately. This usually requires intravenous fluid administration.

If there is no clinical improvement due to emptying of the port system and there is still radiological evidence of slippage (■ Fig. 14.8), the gastric band has to be either removed or repositioned (re-banding).

The slippage of the gastric band can lead to the rare complication of gastric wall necrosis. Clinically, patients present with an acute abdomen. In this case immediate surgical treatment is necessary. The gastric band has to be removed and the necroses resected.

Gastric band migration is an extremely rare complication. Since the pars flaccida technique has been used for the implantation of the gastric band, a rate of less than 1% is assumed. The symptoms of gastric band migration can vary widely, ranging from asymptomatic presentation to severe upper pain with signs of infection. The clinical symptoms may develop slowly.

An infection of the port system may indicate a gastric band migration. For this reason, port infections require further diagnostics.

The diagnosis of gastric band migration is confirmed gastroscopically. The therapy of gastric band migration is the removal of the gastric band. This can be done endoscopically or laparoscopically. If the gastric band can be removed endoscopically, the port system has to be surgically removed simultaneously. This combined procedure should be performed under general anaesthesia. In laparoscopic procedures, the removal of the gastric band can be difficult due to massive adhesions. The gastric band can also be removed by an additional gastrostomy, which is then closed again.

In case of isolated pouch dilatation, the port system is completely emptied. Detailed patient education is necessary to ensure that the patient handles the gastric band appropriately. Particular attention should be paid to small meal sizes to avoid repeated pouch dilatation. It is the task of the obesity surgeons to ensure that the gastric band is filled with an appropriate amount of fluid to prevent that it becomes too tight again.

Esophageal dilatation is often found in combination with gastric pouch dilatation. It is the result of a too tight gastric band in combination with inappropriate eating habits of the patients. Hypomotility of the esophagus is assumed to be an additional cause. Clinical symptoms such as progressive dysphagia, belching, regurgitation and retrosternal pain may be indicative. The diagnosis is confirmed by means of an X-ray after administration of a water-soluble oral contrast medium (pseudo-achalasia) and gastroscopy. First, the port system should be completely drained and, if there is no improvement, the gastric band should be removed.

Dietary lapse can result in a bolus obstruction. Often the food bolus is brought out retrogradely after some time or passes the point of constriction. Rarely, draining of the port system or gastroscopic removal is necessary.

Furthermore, late complications can also be caused by material wear. A frequent material defect is the catheter breakage, which is mainly located next to the junction of the connection tube and the access port. Repair is often achieved simply by shortening the connection tube and reconnecting it to the access port. If the connection tube defect affects the junction with the gastric band, the entire system has to be replaced laparoscopically.

Late Complications After Sleeve Gastrectomy

Late complications after LSG may include stenosis of the gastric sleeve, fistula formation and reflux disease. Stenosis of the gastric sleeve causes nausea, vomiting and dysphagia. As a consequence, exsiccosis may occur. The most frequent anatomical localizations for a stenosis are in the area of the gastroesophageal junction and the incisura angularis. The cause is usually a too small calibration tube or a too wide oversewing of the staple suture line. The diagnosis is made by conventional X-ray with oral contrast medium administration and gastroscopy. Therapy of choice is the temporarily endoscopic implantation of a stent for a period of 4–6 weeks. In contrast to early postoperative stenoses, however, endoscopic balloon dilatation may be considered in the case of late occurring stenoses. If a short segment stenosis cannot be treated sufficiently with these conservative measures, the conversion to a gastric bypass is indicated. If there is a long segment stenosis or if multiple stenoses are present, conversion to a gastric bypass is also recommended.

Similar to acute leaks, late insufficiencies cause pain, malaise and signs of inflammation. The exact aetiology of a late insufficiency is not clear, but often these insufficiencies develop on the basis of ischemia. If late insufficiency is suspected, a CT scan and gastroscopy are performed as in the case of an acute leakage.

Leaks result in abscesses, which are subphrenic and may lead to fistulas. These fistulas often find their way out through the skin, but can also remain intra-abdominal and in rare cases reach the pleura or even the bronchial system. These complications are extremely feared for and may be lethal.

The therapy is the resolution of the insufficiency and the draining of the abscess. Surgical oversewing of the insufficiency is not advisable. The aim of the therapy is initially to "bridge" the insufficiency and sufficient drainage of the abscess formation. In addition to the CT guided drainage of the abscess formation, the insufficiency has to be closed. The implantation of a stent is an option that is used frequently. A stent should not be placed for longer than 6 weeks. Other therapeutic options are vacuum therapy, placement of an "over the scope clip" (OTSC) or endoscopic implantation of a pigtail catheter between the gastric sleeve and the abscess cavity.

A gastroesophageal reflux after LSG occurs in 3–7% of the operated patients. The causes for this are not fully understood yet. A lack of anti-reflux mechanisms is discussed, especially an abolishment of the angle of His. The symptoms of postoperative reflux range from discrete retrosternal burning to regurgitation and nocturnal aspiration. The diagnostic procedure corresponds to the usual reflux diagnostics and includes esophagogastroduodenoscopy, pH test, esophageal manometry and also X-ray diagnostics in head-down position after administration of oral contrast medium. The therapy of reflux is initially symptom-oriented. Proton pump inhibitors are used initially. If the symptoms persist, the conversion to a gastric bypass is recommended (▶ Chap. 15).

Late Complications After Gastric Bypass Surgery

Late anastomotic stenosis of the gastrojejunostomy usually occurs in the first postoperative year and affects about 5% of patients after RYGB surgery. The aetiology of the anastomosis stenosis is not completely understood, possibly chronic tissue ischemia or tensions at the gastrojejunostomy play a causative role. In contrast to early anastomotic stenoses, reports seem to indicate that late stenoses in gastrojejunostomy occur more frequently after usage of circular staplers (21 mm). Symptoms typically include nausea, vomiting, dysphagia and gastroesophageal reflux. Oesophagogastroduodenoscopy (OGD) or gastrointestinal passage X-ray examination with administration of contrast medium are the diagnostic methods of choice; advanced diagnostics by means of CT (with oral contrast medium administration) provides additional information.

Endoscopic balloon dilatation is the therapy of choice and leads to good clinical results in over 90% of cases. Often, however, several dilatations are required at intervals. If an endoscopic dilatation cannot be performed, a surgical creation of a new gastrojejunal anastomosis is necessary. Rarely, anastomosis rupture occurs as a dilation-related complication. In this case a surgical revision is necessary.

14

According to the literature, anastomosis ulcers occur in up to 4% of patients after RYGB surgery. Mostly the anastomosis of the gastrojejunostomy is affected (◨ Fig. 14.9). Etiologically, excessive gastric acid secretion, a too large pouch volume, infection with Helicobacter pylori, chronic insufficient blood supply of the anastomosis, continued nicotine abuse and the intake of non-steroidal anti-inflammatory drugs (NSAID) are suspected. Symptoms are mainly nausea and epigastric pain. Complications may include gastrointestinal blood loss and—rarely—perforation. The diagnosis is confirmed endoscopically by OGD.

Therapeutically, NSAIDs should first be discontinued and proton pump inhibitors (PPI) administered. If the OGD shows evidence of Helicobacter pylori colonisation, eradication therapy is necessary.

In the absence of healing under constant drug therapy or the occurrence of recurrent bleeding, a new gastrojejunostomy has to be applied. If the initially created pouch is large, a reduction of the pouch size should also be considered.

In addition to the gastrojejunal anastomosis stenosis described above postoperative intestinal obstruction may occur more distally. Causes of intestinal obstruction include internal hernias, adhesions, trocar site hernias, stenoses of the jejunojejunostomy and rarely volvulus. The clinical symptoms vary and can be of variable severity. They mainly dependent on the localization of the obstruction. Initially, nausea, vomiting, pain and discomfort are indicative. A complete ileus symptomatology and the clinical picture of an acute abdomen may follow. In most cases an immediate surgical revision is necessary.

Internal hernias after RYGB surgery usually occur in the Peterson's space and next to the enteroenterostomy. They often manifest after weight loss in the second postoperative year. Clinically, the symptoms range from chronic abdominal pain to acute intestinal obstruction. The diagnosis is made by means of CT.

In case of diagnostic uncertainty, exploratory laparoscopy should be indicated generously. The therapy of an internal hernia is always surgical and should initially be started laparoscopically. In case of massive intestinal dilatation or complexity of the surgical site, laparotomy is required. The common channel as well as the biliopancreatic and alimentary loop have to be examined in entirety. The existing herniation and torsion must be resolved. If intestinal damage in the sense of necroses is present, the affected intestinal section has to be resected. Open mesenteric slits or the Peterson's space should be closed with non-resorbable sutures.

Trocar site hernias are rare and occur in dependence of the trocar size. With trocars of 5 mm they practically do not occur. They can cause symptoms similar to those of an internal hernia, the severity of the symptoms also ranges from mild forms to occurrence of an ileus. The surgical therapy includes the repo-

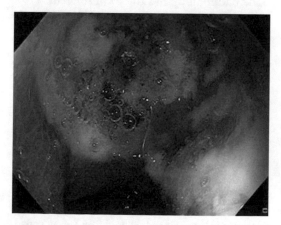

◨ **Fig. 14.9** Gastroscopy and detection of a large anastomosis ulcer

sition of the affected intestinal segments and the closure of the hernia.

It is well known that obesity and also weight loss lead to an increased risk for the formation of gallstones. For this reason, sonographic diagnostics should be performed preoperatively. The frequency with which patients develop cholelithiasis after RYGB surgery varies considerably and is around 10%. Patients with rapid weight loss are particularly at risk.

Patients who are seeking gastric bypass surgery and have symptomatic cholecysto-lithiasis have to undergo a cholecystectomy simultaneously with bariatric surgery. The simultaneous cholecystectomy in patients with symptomless gallstones is discussed controversially. On the one hand, simultaneous cholecystectomy is recommended because of the difficulty of intervention by means of endoscopic retrograde cholangiopancreaticography (ERCP) after gastric bypass surgery, but on the other hand it must be taken into account that simultaneous laparoscopic cholecystectomy leads to an extended length of surgery and thus to an increased surgical risk. Especially in patients with massive steatosis hepatis a simultaneous cholecystectomy is therefore rather discouraged. If necessary, this should then be performed secondarily.

The definition of dumping syndrome after gastric bypass surgery is fuzzy in the literature. In general, it is understood to be a complex of symptoms consisting of abdominal complaints with disturbances of vasomotor function after gastric surgery with loss of pyloric function.

A distinction is made between early dumping occurring immediately postprandially and late dumping with symptoms occurring about 1–3 h after food ingestion.

The cause of early dumping is assumed to be, on the one hand, a pronounced distension of the intestinal wall due to rapid influx of undigested and hyperosmolar food into the alimentary loop and, on the other hand, a pronounced influx of body fluid into the lumen of the small intestine. This results in impaired vasomotor function and even collapse. Clinically, this form of dumping occurs

rarely. In these cases, a too wide gastrojejunal anastomosis is postulated. Therapeutically, a consistent change in diet with a reduced meal size should be aimed at primarily. If the symptoms persist, an attempt to increase the restriction of the anastomosis can be considered. This can be achieved by placing a gastric band around the pouch or by endoscopic procedures (plication in the area of the pouch).

For the so-called late dumping a rapid absorption of simple carbohydrates is reported as causative. This leads to pronounced hyperglycaemia, which is followed by a rapid decline in blood sugar levels leading to symptoms. In addition, however, post-operative changes have to be taken into account, which lead to increased insulin secretion and possibly also to β cell hypertrophy ("nesidioblastosis"). Therefore, the distinction to hyperinsulinemic hypoglycemia syndrome after gastric bypass surgery is blurred and questionable (▶ Sect. 14.8.1).

Blind-loop syndrome is a rare complication after RYGB surgery. Symptoms are flatulence, nausea, abdominal pain and diarrhoea. The cause is assumed to be a bacterial overgrowth of the blind ending loop of the small intestine in the area of the entero-entero-anastomosis. Diagnostically, an H_2-glucose breath test is performed. Before this, however, the presence of fructose or lactose intolerance should be excluded by means of a breath test. Initially, antibiotic therapy is administered; if there is no improvement, resection of the blind ending loop has to be considered.

14.8 Internal Complications

U. Elbelt

In the long term, a deficiency of micro- and macronutrients can occur after bariatric surgery. Hyperinsulinemic hypoglycemia, which occurs after gastric bypass surgery, is challenging to treat. The development of osteoporosis can also lead to a considerable burden of disease, so it should be prevented consequently. After sleeve gastrectomy, reflux symptoms may develop.

In addition to the surgical (mostly) perioperative complications and early postoperative internal complications, which are usually caused by a lack of medication adjustment (such as dehydration, hypokalemia, hypoglycemia, arterial hypotension) or insufficient prophylaxis with medication (cholelithiasis), deficiencies of micro- and macronutrients can lead to health problems (▶ Sect. 14.5). Further complications in the longer term are osteoporosis and (postprandial) hypoglycemia, which can occur after gastric bypass surgery.

14.8.1 Hyperinsulinemic Hypoglycemic Syndrome After Gastric Bypass Surgery

The hypoglycemia occurring in the hyperinsulinemic hypoglycemia syndrome usually leads to hypoglycemia 2–3 h after meals. The symptoms can sometimes be very severe and can extend to a hypoglycemic coma. The hypoglycemia is usually preceded by hyperglycemia caused by food intake. The timing of the onset of this syndrome in the postoperative course is highly variable, and it is not uncommon for symptoms to occur several years after bariatric surgery. The prevalence of a severe form of this syndrome is reported in the literature to be <1% after gastric bypass surgery, while milder forms are much more common (15–70%). The cause is suspected to be increased insulin secretion in β cell hypertrophy ("nesidioblastosis") as a result of postoperatively increased incretin secretion.

According to preliminary results, this pancreatic β cell hyperplasia can be visualized by functional imaging (^{18}F-DOPA-PET, ^{11}C-HTP-PET). Diagnostic algorithms are not established yet. An oral glucose tolerance test (or an alternative mixed-meal test) extended to 5 h with regular measurement of glucose and insulin (in suspected cases of artificial hypoglycemia, also additional measurement of C-peptide) should be performed after careful anamnesis and review of the medication. Therapeutically, for mild forms, a change in diet with smaller sized meals on

a regular basis and the avoidance of carbohydrates with a high glycaemic index is often sufficient. In the case of more severe symptoms, acarbose, calcium antagonists, diazoxide (which is often not tolerated in the long term due to its undesirable effects—in particular its tendency to edema—or somatostatin analogues are administered in the sense of a step-by-step therapy. In cases of hyperinsulinemic hypoglycemia syndrome which cannot be controlled sufficiently by conservative methods, a gastric banding system around the pouch, a resolution of the gastric bypass or a (partial) pancreatectomy should be considered. However, these surgical measures should only be reserved for exceptional cases, as the pronounced symptoms often improve over time.

14.8.2 Osteoporosis

Osteomalacia is a mineralization disorder of newly formed or regenerated bone, usually caused by hypovitaminosis D_3 in combination with calcium deficiency. The resulting secondary hyperparathyroidism further increases bone loss. In contrast, osteoporosis is a reduction in bone density, which is diagnosed by measuring the bone mineral content by means of Dual-X-Ray Absorptiometry (DXA) at the lumbar spine (L1–L4) and/or the proximal femur. From the end of the third decade of life, as we age, there is a decline in bone density with a reduction of bone strength, which is associated with a higher risk of fractures, especially vertebral body fractures and fractures of the proximal femur. If the bone mineral content in postmenopausal women differs by more than −2.5 standard deviations from the mean value of 30-year-old women, osteoporosis is present. This definition can be applied to men over the age of 50. This reduction in bone density is usually referred to as subclinical osteoporosis, and in the presence of osteoporotic fractures as manifest osteoporosis. For brief outline of the clinical approach, the following section does not always differentiate correctly between osteomalacia and osteoporosis.

Usually, prebariatric obese patients have a higher bone density due to the increased body weight (and possibly also due to the increased insulin secretion in the context of insulin resistance and increased leptin levels). In contrast, almost half of the patients already show multifactorial hypovitaminosis D_3 prior to bariatric surgery, and secondary hyperparathyroidism is also common. Calcium deficiency and hypovitaminosis D_3 should, as mentioned, be compensated for preoperatively. The postoperative weight reduction alone leads to a decrease in bone density within the first postoperative year (particularly pronounced in the proximal femur) due to changes in the biomechanical stress on the bone. To what extent this loss of bone density leads to an increased fracture rate in patients undergoing bariatric surgery is not yet clear. However, an increased risk of fractures as well as delayed bone healing can be assumed. Therefore, careful follow-up with prevention of calcium and vitamin D_3 deficiency, repeated information about the preventive relevance of physical activity as well as consistent treatment of secondary hyperparathyroidism are of particular importance. In women in particular, bone density should be measured using the DXA technique prior to the operation. Follow-up monitoring is recommended in the postoperative phase at annual to biennial intervals, depending on the applied guidelines. Drug therapy should be carried out in accordance with the general treatment guidelines, with parenteral administration of pharmaceuticals being favoured.

14.8.3 Further Complications

After sleeve gastrectomy a severe *reflux symptomatology* may occur. A treatment with proton pump inhibitors is often not sufficiently effective. Biliary reflux has to be considered diagnostically. In individual patients, the symptoms can be so severe that the transformation into a gastric bypass has to be made.

A previously clinically inapparent *lactose intolerance* can become manifest postoperatively and leads to complaints. A breath test is performed to confirm the diagnosis. Nutritional advice and a change in diet are recommended.

Acknowledgements We would like to thank Dr. med. Christian Jürgensen, Department of Hepatology and Gastroenterology, Campus Charité Mitte and Campus Virchow-Klinikum, Charité—Universitätsmedizin Berlin, for kindly providing endoscopic images and Prof. Dr. med. Jörg-Wilhelm Oestmann, Department of Radiology (including Pediatric Radiology), Charité—Universitätsmedizin Berlin, for the radiological findings provided.

References

14.1–14.3

Dieckmann S (2013) Ernährung nach Magenbypassoperation, 2. Aufl. WiKu-Wissenschaftsverlag Dr. Stein, Köln & Duisburg

Handzlik-Orlik G, Holecki M, Orlik B, et al. (2014) Nutrition management of post-bariatric surgery patient. Nutr Clin Pract, XX(X): 1–10

Hellbardt M (Hrsg) (2013) Ernährung im Kontext der bariatrischen Chirurgie, 4. Aufl. Pabst Science Publishers, Lengerich Berlin Bremen Miami Riga Viernheim Wien Zagreb

Moizé V, Pi-Sunyer X, Mochari H et al (2010) Nutritional pyramid for post-gastric bypass patients. Obes Surg 20:1133–1141. Springer Science+Business Media

Saltzmann E, Karl P (2013) Nutrient deficiencies after gastric bypass surgery. Ann Rev Nutr 33:183–203

14.7.1

Gagner M, Buchwald JN (2014) Comparison of laparoscopic sleeve gastrectomy leak rates in four staple-line reinforcement options: a systematic review. Surg Obes Relat Dis 10:713–723

Parikh M, Issa R, McCrillis A, Saunders JK et al (2013) Surgical strategies that may decrease leak after laparoscopic sleeve gastrectomy. A systematic review and meta-analysis of 9991 cases. Ann Surg 257: 231–237

Further Readings

14.1–14.3

Stein J, Stier C, Raab H et al (2014) Review article: the nutritional and pharmacological consequences of obesity surgery. Aliment Pharmacol Ther 40:582–609

14.4

Deutsche Gesellschaft für Allgemein- und Viszeral-chirurgie, Chirurgische Arbeitsgemeinschaft für Adipositastherapie (CAADIP), Deutsche Adipositas-Gesellschaft (DAAG), Deutsche Gesellschaft für Psychosomatische Medizin und Psychotherapie, Deutsche Gesellschaft für Ernährungsmedizin (2010) S3-Leitlinie: Chirurgie der Adipositas. http://www.adipositas-gesellschaft.de/fileadmin/PDF/Leitlinien/ADIP-6-2010.pdf. (Letzter Zugriff: 25. April 2016)

Gould JC et al (2007) Impact of routine and long term follow up on weight loss after laparoscopic gastric bypass. Surger Obes Relat Dis 3:627–630

Harper J et al (2007) What happens to patients who do not follow-up after bariatric surgery? Am Surg 73:181–184

Sauerland S, Angrisani L, Belachew M et al (2005) Obesity surgery. Evidence-based guidelines of the European Association for Endoscopic Surgery. Surg Endosc 19:200–221

14.5

Bender G, Allolio B (2010) Welche Bedeutung hat die Nachsorge nach bariatrischer Chirurgie? J Klin Endokrinol Stoffw 3:12–16

Chirurgische Arbeitsgemeinschaft für Adipositasthera-pie, Deutsche Adipositas-Gesellschaft, Deutsche Gesellschaft für Psychosomatische Medizin und Psy-chotherapie, Deutsche Gesellschaft für Ernährungs-medizin (2010) S-3 Leitlinie: Chirurgie der Adipositas. http://www.adipositas-gesellschaft.de/fileadmin/PDF/Leitlinien/ADIP-6-2010.pdf. (Letz-ter Zugriff: 25. April 2016)

Deutsche Adipositas-Gesellschaft, Deutsche Diabetes Gesellschaft, Deutsche Gesellschaft für Ernährung, Deutsche Gesellschaft für Ernährungsmedizin (2014) Interdisziplinäre Leitlinie der Qualität S3 zur "Prävention und Therapie der Adipositas". AWMF-Register Nr. 050/001. Klasse: S3 Version 2.0

Fried M, Yumuk V, Oppert J-M et al (2013) Interdisci-plinary European giudelines on metabolic and barit-ric surgery. Obes Facts 6:449–468

Hellbardt M (Hrsg) (2011) Ernährung im Kontext der bariatrischen Chirurgie, 1. Aufl. Pabst Science Pub-lishers, Lengerich

Herpertz S (2015) Sollen/müssen wir die Behandlung der Adipositas den Chirurgen überlassen? Psychother Psych Med 65:42–44

Lammert F, Neubrand MW, Bittner R et al (2007) S-3 Leitlinie der Deutschen Gesellschaft für Verdauungs- und Stoffwechselkrankheiten und der Deutschen Gesellschaft für Viszeralchirurgie zur Diagnostik und Behandlung von Gallensteinen. AWMF-Regis-ter-Nr. 021/008. Z Gastroenterol 45:971–1001

Malinowski SS (2006) Nutritional and metabolic com-plications of bariatric surgery. Am J Med Sci 331: 219–225

Mechanik JI, Youdim A, Jones DB et al (2013) Clinical practice guidelines for the perioperative nutritional, metabolic, and nonsurgical support of the bariatric surgery patient-2013 update: cosponsored by Ameri-can Association of Clinical Endocrinologists, The Obesity Society, and American Society for Metabolic & Bariatric Surgery. Obesity 21:S1–S27

Padwal R, Brocks D, Sharma AM (2009) A systematic review of drug absorption following bariatric surgery and its theoretical implications. Obes Rev 11:41–50. https://doi.org/10.1111/j.1467-789X.2009.00614.x

Schultes B, Thurnheer M (2012) Bariatrische Chirurgie. Diabetologie 7:R17–R36

Soleymani T, Tejavanija S, Morgan S (2011a) Obesity, bariatric surgery, and bone. Curr Opin Rheumatol 23:396–405

Tindle HA, Omalu B, Courcoulas A et al (2010) Risk of suicide after long-term follow-up from bariatric sur-gery. Am J Med 123:1036–1042

14.6

Herpertz S, Müller A, Burgmer R, Crosby RD, de Zwaan M, Legenbauer T (2015) Health-related quality of life and psychological functioning 9 years after restrictive surgical treatment for obesity. Surg Obes Relat Dis 11:1361–1370. https://doi.org/10.1016/j.soard.2015.04.008

Karmali S, Brar B, Shi X, Sharma AM, de Gara C, Birch DW (2013) Weight recidivism post-bariatric surgery: a systematic review. Obes Surg 23:1922–1933

Rudolph A, Hilbert A (2013) Post-operative behavioural management in bariatric surgery: a systematic review and meta-analysis of randomized controlled trials. Obes Rev 14:292–302

Sheets CS, Peat CM, Berg KC et al (2015) Post-operative psychosocial predictors of outcome in bariatric sur-gery. Obes Surg 25:330–345

Wimmelmann CL, Dela F, Mortensen EL (2014) Psycho-logical predictors of weight loss after bariatric sur-gery: a review of the recent research. Obes Res Clin Pract 8:e299–e313

14.7.1

Ablanopoulos K, Alevizos L, Flessas J et al (2012) Rein-forcing the staple line during laparoscopic sleeve gastrectomy: prospective randomized clinical study comparing 2 different techniques: preliminary results. Obes Surg 22:42–46

Bernante P, Francini Pesenti F, Toniato A et al (2005) Obstructive symptoms associated with the 9.75-cm Lap-Band in the first 24 hours using the pars flaccida approach. Obes Surg 15:357–360

Bingham J, Shawhan R, Parker R, Wigboldy J, Sohn V (2015) Computed tomography scan versus upper gastrointestinal fluoroscopy for diagnosis of staple line leak following bariatric surgery. Am J Surg 209: 810–814

D'Ugo S, Gentileschi P, Benavoli D et al (2014) Compara-tive use of different techniques for leak and bleeding prevention during laparoscopic sleeve gastrectomy: a multicenter study. Surg Obes Relat Dis 10:450–454

Favretti F, Cadiere GB, Segato G et al (1997) Laparoscopic adjustable silicone gastric banding (Lap-Band®): how to avoid complications. Obes Surg 7:352–358

Fernandez AZ, DeMaria EJ, Tichansky DS et al (2004) Experience with over 3000 open and laparoscopic bariatric procedures: multivariate analysis of factors related to leak and resultant mortality. Surg Endos 18:193–197

Fischer A, Bausch D, Richter-Schraq HJ (2013) Use of a specially designed partially covered self-expandable metal stent (PSEMS) with a 40-mm diameter for the treatment of upper gastrointestinal suture or staple line leaks in 11 cases. Surg Endosc 27:642–647

Heneghan HM, Meron-Eldar S, Yenumula P et al (2012) Incidence and management of bleeding complications after gastric bypass surgery in the morbidly obese. Surg Obes Relat Dis 8:729–735

Nguyen NT, Herta S, Gelfand D et al (2004) Bowel obstruction after laparoscopic Roux-en-Y gastric bypass. Obes Surg 14:190–196

Rabl C, Peeva S, Prado K et al (2011) Early and late abdominal bleeding after Rou-en-Y gastric bypass: sources and tailored therapeutic strategies. Obes Surg 21:413–420

Sakran N, Goitein D, Raziel A et al (2013) Gastric leaks after sleeve gastrectomy: a multicenter experience with 2834 patients. Surg Endosc 27:240–250

Sarkhosh K, Birch DW, Sharma A, Karmali S (2013) Complications associated with laparoscopic sleeve gastrectomy for morbid obesity: a surgeon's guide. Can J Surg 56:347–352

Schiesser M, Kressig P, Bueter M et al (2014) Successful endoscopic management of gastrointestinal leakages after laparoscopic Roux-en-Y gastric bypass surgery. Dig Surg 31:67–70

14.7.2

Barba CA, Butensky MS, Lorenzo M, Newman R (2003) Endoscopic dilation of gastroesophageal anastomosis stricture after gastric bypass. Surg Endosc 17:416–420

Chevallier JM, Zinzindohoue F, Douard R et al (2004) Complications after laparoscopic adjustable gastric banding for morbid obesity: experience with 1000 patients over 7 years. Obes Surg 14:407–414

Hainaux B, Agneessens E, Rubesova E et al (2005) Intragastric band erosion after laparoscopic adjustable gastric banding for morbid obesity: imaging characteristics of an underreported complication. Am J Roentgenol 184:109–112

Hamad GG, Ikramuddin S, Gourash WF, Schauer PR (2003) Elective cholecystectomy during laparoscopic Roux-en-Y gastric bypass: is it worth the wait? Obes Surg 13:76–81

Hendricks LS, Alvarenga E, Dhanabalsamy N et al (2015) Impact of sleeve gastrectomy on gastroesophageal reflux disease in a morbidly obese population undergoing bariatric surgery. Surg Obes Relat Dis 12:511–517

Husain S, Ahmed AR, Johnson J, Boss T, O'Malley W (2007) Small-bowel obstruction after laparoscopic Roux-en-Y gastric bypass: etiology, diagnosis, and management. Arch Surg 142:988–993

Langer FB, Bohdjalian A, ShakeriLidenmühler S, Schoppmann SF, Zacherl J, Prager G (2010) Conversion from sleeve gastrectomy to Roux-en-Y gastric bypass–indications and outcome. Obes Surg 20:835–840

Paroz A, Calmes JM, Giusti V, Suter M (2006) Internal hernia after laparoscopic Roux-en-Y gastric bypass for morbid obesity: a continuous challenge in bariatric surgery. Obes Surg 16:1482–1487

Ponce J, Fromm R, Paynter J (2006) Outcomes after laparoscopic adjustable gastric band repositioning for slippage or pouch dilation. Surg Obes Relat Dis 2:627–631

Sammour T, Hill AG, Singh P, Ranasinghe A, Babor R, Rahman H (2010) Laparoscopic sleeve gastrectomy as a single-stage bariatric procedure. Obes Surg 20:271–275

Seyfried F, Wierlemann A, Bala M, Fassnacht M, Jurowich C (2015) Dumping syndrome: diagnostics and therapeutic options. Chirurg 86:847–854

Silecchia G, Restuccia A, Elmore U et al (2001) Laparoscopic adjustable silicone gastric banding: prospective evaluation of intragastric migration of the lap-band. Surg Laparosc Endosc Percutan Tech 11:229–234

Spivak H, Rubin M (2003) Laparoscopic management of lap-band slippage. Obes Surg 13:116–120

Tran D, Rhoden DH, Cacchione RN, Baldwin L, Allen JW (2004) Techniques for repair of gastric prolapse after laparoscopic gastric banding. J Laparoendosc Adv Surg Tech A 14:117–120

14.8

De Heide LJM, Glaudemans AWJM, Oomen PHN et al (2012) Functional imaging in hyperinsulinemic hypoglycemia after gastric bypass surgery for morbid obesity. JCEM 97:E963–E967

De Heide LJM, Laskewitz AJ, Apers JA (2014) Treatment of severe postRYGB hyperinsulinemic hypoglycemia with pasireotide: a comparison with octrotide on insulin, glucagon, and GLP-1. Surg Obes Relat Dis 10:e31–e33

Halperin F, Goldfine AB (2013) Metabolic surgery for type 2 diabetes: efficacy and risks. Curr Opin Endocrinol Diabetes Obes 20:98–105

Soleymani T, Tejavanija S, Morgan S (2011b) Obesity, bariatric surgery, and bone. Curr Opin Rheumatol 23:396–405

14

Revision and Redo Operations After Bariatric Procedures

T. Dziodzio and C. Denecke

Contents

© Springer-Verlag GmbH Germany, part of Springer Nature 2022
J. Ordemann, U. Elbelt (eds.), *Obesity and Metabolic Surgery*,
https://doi.org/10.1007/978-3-662-63227-7_15

15.1 Background

Bariatric surgery is now an established and long-term successful therapeutic option in the treatment of morbid obesity and associated concomitant diseases. With the increasing number of primary interventions, the number of revision and redo interventions after bariatric surgery is also increasing worldwide.

The term "revision surgery" is usually used as a generic term for renewed operations for the therapy of procedure-specific complications or in the case of therapy failure of the primary bariatric procedure. The term "redo", on the other hand, refers to the conversion of a bariatric procedure into another bariatric procedure.

Due to the different surgical techniques used in primary procedure (adjustable gastric banding, gastric tube, gastric bypass and now abandoned procedures such as vertical gastroplasty), the bariatric surgeon is confronted with different patient complaints and various complications. The most frequent indication for a redo procedure is the so-called "therapy failure", however a clear definition is missing. In most cases, this refers to patients who have not lost weight after the primary procedure or who have regained weight.

Since the causes are usually multifactorial, comprehensive diagnostics in a specialized center needs to be performed before the indication for a revision/redo procedure. In addition to functional diagnostics by means of endoscopy and imaging procedures (upper gastrointestinal series), the patient's nutritional behaviour and a psychosomatic state should be examined to exclude non-surgical causes. Revision/redo procedure should be postponed until a non-surgical cause is treated or addressed. In the case of patients who have already undergone multiple surgeries, diagnostics can be extended by a computed tomography.

The decision to perform and the choice of the appropriate revision/redo intervention must be carefully considered. It must ultimately be made after an individual consultation with the patient, taking into account the patient's symptoms, psychological stress, chances of success and surgical risk.

15.2 Revision/Redo Procedure After Gastric Banding

The low perioperative complication rate and the effective short-term weight reduction led to the widespread use of the gastric banding, especially around the turn of the millennium. In the long term, however, a high rate of band failure was observed in up to 50% of patients requiring a revision/redo surgery. The high rate of late complications and band failure is the reason for the worldwide decline in the use of gastric banding surgeries. While in 2003 the gastric banding system was still the most common bariatric procedure in Germany (>50% of all bariatric procedures) it is now in third place, while gastric bypass and sleeve gastrectomy currently account for 95% of the bariatric procedures performed in Germany. However, the initial widespread use of this procedure has led to the situation that even today many patients with band failure or band complications are seeking a redo/revision procedure.

15.2.1 Indication

Patients after gastric band implantation can have different complaints and complications. Patient's symptoms are the main factor for decision making on an adequate surgical therapy (band removal/conversion surgery). In addition, gastric banding can lead to material-related or technical complications, such as band leakage or port-site infections, and surgical complications, such as band slippage and band migration (see also ▶ Sect. 14.7).

> **Practical Tip**
>
> A revision procedure with refixation of the gastric band or re-banding should only be performed if adequate weight loss has been achieved by the gastric band implantation and no additional functional complaints are present.

On the other hand, patients who have not achieved adequate weight reduction before the onset of band dysfunction or patients with functional complaints should be advised to undergo conversion surgery (redo). Since the long-term success of the gastric band appears uncertain, re-banding or refixation surgery should always be critically reviewed and the patient should be informed about surgical alternatives.

15.2.2 Procedure

The advantage of a refixation of the gastric band or a re-banding is the short operation time and the integrity of the anatomy. In addition, if symptoms occur, there is still the possibility of band removal and the complete reversibility of the procedure. Gastric banding explantation is indicated for patients with functional complaints due to band dysfunction (slippage, band erosion) or in case of therapy failure. Depending on the complication, the gastric band can be removed laparoscopically, open surgically or combined laparoscopically/endoscopically (in case of complete band migration).

Since weight regain almost always occurs after band removal, the patient should be recommended a conversion procedure. The most common conversion operations are the laparoscopic sleeve gastrectomy and the laparoscopic gastric bypass surgery. Several factors play a role in decision making for the right conversion surgery. In cases with therapy failure due to the high-calorie food intake ("sweet eater"), the use of a sleeve gastrectomy should be carefully considered, as in this case sufficient weight loss is rarely achieved. These patients are more likely to benefit from a gastric bypass surgery due to its malabsorptive effects.

After determination of the conversion therapy, it is necessary to decide whether the conversion should be carried out in a one-step or in two-step approach. In observational studies the complication rate—particularly with regard to leakage—were observed slightly higher in single-stage procedures. Therefore, some authors recommend to perform single-step procedures only if the surgical site is inconspicuous and to generously provide the indication for a two-step procedure at an interval of 2–4 months if there are signs of surgical site inflammation or the band removal is difficult.

Practical Tip

When removing the band, always ensure that the band channel is completely split and a partial resection of the fibrous channel is performed to achieve a complete re-expansion of the stomach and to restore the preoperative anatomy.

The band removal is performed via the former trocar sites in the upper abdomen. After creation of the capnoperitoneum, exploration and adhesiolysis, the left lobe of the liver is first lifted and the port tube identified. The port tube is the leading structure to the gastric band. After visualization of the band, the overlying fundus cuff is mobilized, the angle of His is identified and the fibrous capsule around the ligament is detached. Once the band is exposed, it can be opened at the band lock. The band and port chamber are then removed. In case of a subsequent revision bypass operation (surgical technique ▶ Chap. 10), the formation of anastomosis in the area of the former fibrous canal should be avoided, as the risk of anastomosis insufficiency might be increased.

15.3 Revision/Redo Procedure After Sleeve Gastrectomy

Sleeve gastrectomy is one of the most common bariatric procedures worldwide and is almost comparable to gastric bypass surgery in terms of short-term weight loss and amelioration of obesity-related diseases. Albeit, sleeve gastrectomy results in lower morbidity and mortality compared to the gastric bypass surgery, patients after sleeve gastrectomy suffer more frequently from gastroesophageal reflux. Furthermore, long-term weight reduction is less pronounced compared to gastric bypass surgery due to gradual sleeve dilation, hormonal adaption, and recurrence of improper eating behaviours.

15.3.1 Indication

Similar to the gastric banding, insufficient weight loss can occur after sleeve gastrectomy. The reason for this can be a lack of restriction due to a too large sleeve tube after primary surgery or a high-calorie diet ("sweet-eater"). In addition, gradual sleeve dilation can occur—especially if the fundus is left partially intact—with consecutive weight regain.

Insufficient weight loss and regain of weight regain are the most frequent indications for a revision/redo procedure after gastrectomy. Functional complaints such as a PPI-resistant reflux gastroesophageal reflux can also be an indication for a revisional procedure. Careful diagnostics and examination of the medical history are necessary for planning and indication of redo or conversion procedure.

> **Practical Tip**
>
> It is very important to carefully considered whether the patient benefits from a revisional restrictive procedure or rather from a malabsorptive procedure.

15.3.2 Procedure

Two procedures play a decisive role in the therapy of sleeve gastrectomy failure:

In case of therapy failure due to sleeve dilatation and in patients without gastroesophageal reflux a revisional sleeve gastrectomy can be considered. This operation is performed in a similar way to the primary intervention. The restriction is restored by resection and reshaping of the dilated gastric sleeve. The advantages of this method are the short operation time and the manageability of the procedure. However, known technical disadvantages such as insufficiencies, strictures and stenosis need to be considered. In case of "sweet-eater" patients, the indication for a redo of a restrictive procedure should be critically evaluated. In exceptional cases, such as older patients or patients with severe multimorbidity, the implementation of a POSE procedure (▶ Sect. 18.2) may be considered as an alternative to the sleeve gastrectomy. The surgical access is performed via the former trocar sites in the upper abdomen. After application of the capnoperitoneum, exploration and adhesiolysis of the neo-greater curvature of the stomach is performed. Then the gastric sleeve is measured in the already described way (▶ Chap. 9). It is important to resect the remaining fundus.

In patients with gastroesophageal reflux or in patients with sleeve failure without sleeve dilatation the conversion into a gastric bypass should be performed. Although this malabsorptive procedure is associated with a higher rate of perioperative complications, it can lead to sufficient weight loss, especially in patients with high-caloric dietary habits.

> **Practical Tip**
>
> The conversion of a sleeve gastrectomy to a gastric bypass needs to be performed carefully to ensure a tissue-sparing preparation and to keep a sufficient safety distance from the staple suture line of the gastric sleeve in order maintain adequate perfusion of the newly created anastomosis.

Another possibility for redo intervention is the creation of an omega loop bypass (▶ Sect. 11.1).

15.4 Revision/Redo Procedure After Gastric Bypass Surgery

Roux-en-Y gastric bypass is the most common bariatric procedure worldwide and is considered the gold standard of bariatric surgery with the best-proven effectiveness and sustainability in terms of weight reduction and amelioration of obesity-related diseases. Due to different surgical techniques of the stapler anastomoses (linear or circular),

15

different lengths of the alimentary and biliopancreatic limbs as well as different pouch sizes, various complications can occur, requiring revision/redo procedures. In addition, eating disorders can lead to dilatation of the pouch, anastomosis and/or the alimentary limb.

15.4.1 Indication

The most common cause of a revision/redo procedure is inadequate weight loss or weight regain. Up to 35% of patients are affected by inadequate weight loss after gastric bypass in the long-term follow-up due to a malfunction of the restrictive components of the gastric bypass (e.g., excessively large stomach pouch during primary surgery or acquired pouch dilatation). In addition to the pouch size, the diameter of the gastrojejunostomy may also play a decisive role in weight regain. Additionally, a tight anastomosis can lead to pouch dilatation if patients with disturbed eating habits.

Anastomosis ulcers can also lead to scarring of the anastomosis ring and cause pouch dilatation. A too wide anastomosis, on the other hand, can lead to a dilation of the alimentary limb causing a reservoir and acting as a neo-stomach. Only after ruling out a dilatation of the pouch and the alimentary limb by imaging and endoscopic diagnosis, the surgical expansion of the malabsorptive components can be considered. However, a careful assessment of deficiency symptoms should be carried out first. Less frequent indications for a revision/redo procedure are functional complaints such as dumping syndrome or—very rarely—persistent gastroesophageal reflux.

15.4.2 Procedure

In case of therapy failure, conversion operations after gastric bypass surgery play a subordinate role and are only performed in exceptional situations. Revision/redo procedures after gastric bypass surgery are usually very complex procedures with a high compli-

cation rates. They should therefore only be performed by experienced surgeons in specialized bariatric centers.

The most common cause of therapy failure after gastric bypass is caused by stomach pouch size and the width of the gastrojejunostomy. If pouch dilatation has been diagnosed, the goal of the redo procedure is pouch size reduction by resection of the stomach pouch and repositioning of the gastrojejunostomy. More rarely, the creation of a gastric band (band-over-bypass, salvage banding) can also support the restrictive function (▶ Sect. 18.5). This supporting anastomosis ring is associated with the same risk factors as gastric banding. Especially for the revision of the anastomosis and for reshaping of the pouch, the Apollo overstitch™ has been established as a gentle endoscopic method especially for patients with a high perioperative risk. With this method, the reduction of the stomach is carried out via intragastral endoscopic access by suturing the large curvature.

In patients with inconspicuous pouch and anastomosis ratios, a distal shift of the Roux-en-Y anastomosis can lead to an increase of the malabsorptive component and an adequate weight reduction. However, a too deep Roux-en-Y anastomosis can promote complaints such as dumping and deficiency symptoms.

The operative access for the revision gastric bypass is performed via the former trocar sites in the upper abdomen. Due to varying degrees of adhesions, conversion to open access is often necessary. After exploration and adhesiolysis, a revision of the gastric pouch, Roux-en-Y anastomosis or a combination of both is performed. In rare cases a biliopancreatic diversion with duodenal switch may be indicated.

In cases with pronounced functional complaints after gastric bypass surgery, a reverse operation to the original anatomy is possible. However, this procedure is extremely complex and only justified in exceptional cases. In addition, the restoration of the original anatomical conditions may not always be accompanied by original functionality due to adhesions and scarring.

Further Readings

Alvarez V, Carrasco F, Cuevas A, Valenzuela B, Muñoz G, Ghiardo D et al (2016) Mechanisms of long-term weight regain in patients undergoing sleeve gastrectomy. Nutrition 32:303–308

Angrisani L, Santonicola A, Iovino P, Formisano G, Buchwald H, Scopinaro N (2015) Bariatric surgery worldwide 2013. Obes Surg 25:1822–1832

Buchwald H, Oien DM (2013) Metabolic/bariatric surgery worldwide 2011. Obes Surg 23:427–436

Fischer L, Wekerle A-L, Bruckner T, Wegener I, Diener MK, Frankenberg MV et al (2015) BariSurg trial: Sleeve gastrectomy versus Roux-en-Y gastric bypass in obese patients with BMI 35–60 kg/m(2)—a multi-centre randomized patient and observer blind non-inferiority trial. BMC Surg 15:87

Gadiot RPM, Biter LU, van Mil S, Zengerink HF, Apers J, Mannaerts GHH (2016) Long-term results of laparoscopic sleeve gastrectomy for morbid obesity: 5 to 8-year results. Obes Surg. 2016 May 14 (Epub ahead of print). www.ncbi.nlm.nih.gov/pubmed/27178407. (05.07.2016)

Kumar N (2015) Endoscopic therapy for weight loss: Gastroplasty, duodenal sleeves, intragastric balloons, and aspiration. World J Gastrointest Endosc 7:847–859

Kuzminov A, Palmer AJ, Wilkinson S, Khatsiev B, Venn AJ (2016) Re-operations after secondary bariatric surgery: a systematic review. Obes Surg 26(9):2237–2247. https://doi.org/10.1007/s11695-016-2252-7. 2016 Jun 8 (Epub ahead of print). www.ncbi.nlm.nih.gov/pubmed/27272668 (05.07.2016)

Stroh C, Weiner R, Wolff S, Knoll C, Manger T (2015a) Revisional surgery and reoperations in obesity and metabolic surgery: data analysis of the German bariatric surgery registry 2005–2012. Chirurg 86(4):346–354

Stroh C, Weiner R, Wolff S, Lerche C, Knoll C, Keller T et al (2015b) One versus two-step Roux-en-Y gastric bypass after gastric banding—data analysis of the German Bariatric Surgery Registry. Obes Surg 25:755–762

Tran DD, Nwokeabia ID, Purnell S, Zafar SN, Ortega G, Hughes K et al (2016) Revision of Roux-En-Y gastric bypass for weight regain: a systematic review of techniques and outcomes. Obes Surg 26:1627–1634

Vijgen GHEJ, Schouten R, Bouvy ND, Greve JWM (2012) Salvage banding for failed Roux-en-Y gastric bypass. Surg Obes Relat Dis 8:803–808

15

Special Patient Groups in Bariatric Surgery

J. Mühlsteiner, P. Stauch, and T. P. Hüttl

Contents

© Springer-Verlag GmbH Germany, part of Springer Nature 2022
J. Ordemann, U. Elbelt (eds.), *Obesity and Metabolic Surgery*,
https://doi.org/10.1007/978-3-662-63227-7_16

16.1 Surgery at Older Age

The federal health report for Germany shows an increase in the body mass index of older people over the last few years. The proportion of the population with a BMI > 30 kg/m² rose from 18.9% in 1999 to 21.9% in 2013, and the proportion of people over 70 years of age with a BMI > 30 kg/m² also increased significantly from 14.5% to 20.3%.

Derived from these data and with additionally increasing life expectancy, obesity surgery is also gaining importance for older patients. In the current S3 guideline of obesity surgery (2010), the previously recommended upper age limit of 65 years of life has already been withdrawn without specifying a new upper limit.

Age alone is therefore no longer a contraindication to bariatric surgery. So far, there is no scientifically defined upper age limit. Thus, the general condition and the comorbidities of the individual patient are increasingly becoming the focus of attention. Preoperatively, frequent comorbidities of obesity such as diabetes mellitus type 2, cardiovascular diseases and orthopaedic limitations have to be assessed carefully. In particular, the presence of underlying diseases associated with a catabolic state such as neoplasm and advanced liver disease has to be excluded in older patients.

The reduction or remission of already advanced comorbidities is rarely the primary indication for surgery in older patients. Rather, immobility and the need for care can be avoided by weight loss. The maintained or regained independence, participation in social life through increased mobility and physical performance significantly improve the quality of life.

With regard to the literature on choice of the surgical procedure, no clear recommendation can be made at this point. In a study by Musella et al. (2014), which compares the implantation of a gastric band and sleeve gastrectomy, a similarly weight loss and a reduction in comorbidities could be demonstrated after a 5-year follow-up period with a comparable perioperative risk for both surgical procedures. Sugerman et al. (2004) show in a retrospective study that gastric bypass surgery leads to the highest and most effective weight loss in older patients.

In general, the long-term weight loss achieved in older patients who have undergone surgery is less than that achieved in patients who have undergone surgery at a younger age. This could be shown in a prospective comparative study between older and younger patients undergoing gastric bypass surgery. Huang and Garg (2015) retrospectively compared their results in laparoscopically performed Roux-en-Y-bypass (LRYGB) with sleeve gastrectomy. Again, both procedures showed positive effects on comorbidities. However, morbidity and revision rate were increased in patients with LRYGB. The laparoscopic mini-bypass seems to be promising as a technically simple and safe surgical procedure with a low complication rate also in terms of weight loss and reduction of comorbidities in older patients. In a retrospective analysis of Roux-en-Y-bypasses a 30-day mortality of 0.7% could be demonstrated in patients over 60 years of age. A similarly high mortality rate (0.7% for sleeve gastrectomy and 0.5% for Roux-en-Y-bypass) was shown in another large-scale study by Qin and Luo (2014). No statistically significant difference could be detected between surgical and immediate postoperative complications. In the long term, sleeve gastrectomy is the safer surgical method according to this study.

> **Practical Tip**
>
> In conclusion, increased age does not represent a risk factor of its own for bariatric surgery, but rather internal comorbidities must be taken into account.

16.2 Surgery in Childhood and Adolescence

The prevalence of childhood and adolescent obesity has increased significantly in recent years, both in Germany and worldwide. Today, increased body weight is the most common diet-related health disorder among children and adolescents in Germany. Depending on the definition, 10–20% of all school children and adolescents in Germany are overweight. In addition, the number of extremely obese adolescents has risen significantly.

The burden of obesity, especially in this age group, results from functional limitation as well as psychosocial impairment. Furthermore, children and adolescents with obesity show a higher comorbidity than their normal weight counterparts and a significantly increased risk of morbidity and mortality in adulthood. The health risks of obesity in adulthood are scientifically well documented, whereby the manifestation of obesity in childhood has an additional unfavourable influence. Due to the propagated ideal of beauty, obese adolescents are often stigmatized. This can lead to a reduced self-esteem, disturbs the psychosocial development and possibly also promotes the development of eating disorders.

It could be shown that the BMI is a sufficient measure of total body fat mass. As this applies not only to adults but also to children and adolescents, both the Childhood Group of the International Obesity Task Force (IOTF) and the European Childhood Obesity Group (ECOG) recommend the use of the BMI to define overweight and obesity in children and adolescents. Since the BMI in childhood and adolescence is influenced by well-defined age- and gender-specific characteristics in accordance with the physiological changes in the percentage body fat mass, age and gender must be taken into account for its assessment. Individual BMI values can be assessed using population-specific reference values for childhood and adolescence (in the form of age- and gender-specific percentiles, ◘ Fig. 16.1). The definition of overweight or obesity and extreme obesity should be based on the 90th or 97th and 99.5th percentiles, respectively, in an age- and gender-specific manner (◘ Table 16.1).

In addition to clinical and laboratory diagnostics, a genetic testing is also required in cases of suspicion, as certain genetic diseases may be associated with obesity (see also ▶ Sect. 5.2). Initial indications of somatic secondary diseases such as hypertension, lipid metabolism disorders, diabetes mellitus type 2 or disorders of orthopaedic issues must be taken into account. It is always necessary to consult a child and adolescent psychiatrist. The younger a patient is, the more important is the co-treatment by the paediatrician.

Children and adolescents with chronic diseases or with mental disabilities are more often overweight and obese. Obesity in these children and adolescents is a major risk factor for the deterioration of the underlying disability.

The risk of dying of an obesity-related disease increases by 6–7% every 2 years that the child or adolescent suffers from obesity. Obesity in children and adolescents should therefore be treated early and effectively.

Preventive measures to avoid obesity play a decisive role. Although the primarily conservative therapy has good short-term success, the long-term results are often disappointing. A Cochrane analysis showed an average weight loss of 1.7 kg/m^2 BMI after 12 months.

Bariatric surgery in adolescence leads to significant weight loss and remission of obesity-specific comorbidities such as diabetes mellitus type 2, arterial hypertension and sleep apnea. In addition, psychological stabilization often occurs.

There are already reports of the successful use of surgical measures to treat extreme overweight in adolescents from the 1970s and 1980s. Surgery already in childhood is still controversially discussed. The youngest child to have undergone bariatric surgery published to date was a 2.5-year-old boy weighing 33 kg with a BMI of 41.1 kg/m^2. After exclusion of endocrinological causes and exhaustion of the "conservative" therapy, a laparoscopic sleeve gastrectomy was performed on him. In a postoperative observation period of 2.5 years, a weight loss to 24 kg (BMI 24 kg/m^2) occurred.

Currently, the guidelines of the "International Pediatric Endosurgery Group" (IPEG) stipulate that surgical intervention should be considered in adolescents with a BMI > 40 kg/m^2 or a BMI > 35 kg/m^2 with severe comorbidities when the patients are nearly fully-grown and conservative treatment methods have failed. This guideline is

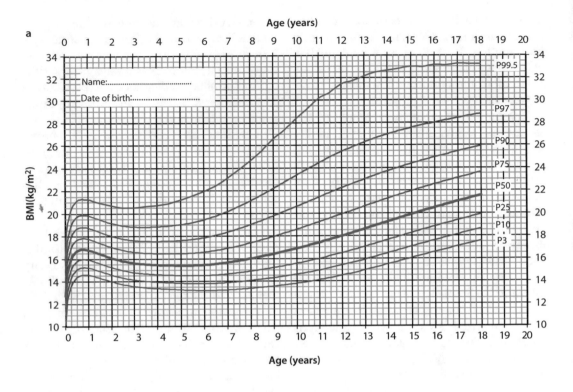

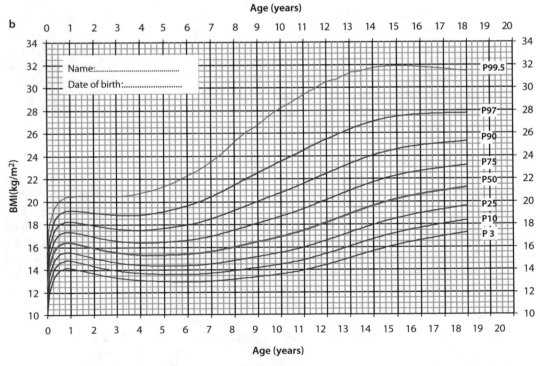

□ Fig. 16.1 Gender and age-specific BMI percentiles for children and adolescents. **a** Boys, **b** girls. (From Wabitsch 2014, modified according to Kromeyer-Hauschild et al. 2001)

◻ Table 16.1 Definition of overweight and obesity in childhood and adolescence

Overweight	BMI percentile > 90–97
Obesity	BMI percentile > 97–99.5
Extreme obesity	BMI percentile > 99.5

based on a meta-analysis by Treadwell et al. (2008). Corresponding recommendations are also considered in international guidelines. A joint decision-making process involving the paediatrician, the surgeon, the behavioural therapist as well as the patient and his parents is essential, as patients under 18 years of age require parental consent and the patient himself can only partially assume responsibility. Furthermore, the surgical procedure should be performed in specialised centres with expertise and the presence of a multidisciplinary team (each of which is a specialist in childhood obesity therapy). Potential long-term side effects or complications of a bariatric surgical procedure in childhood and adolescence, especially with regard to physical and mental development, cannot be excluded with certainty at the current state of research; adolescents and their custodians should be made aware of this risk, which cannot be further specified.

Furthermore, a long-term concept for the care of the patient has to be available beyond the intervention. The willingness of the patient and his family to take part in postoperative aftercare on a long-term basis is also necessary.

In principle, the same surgical procedures as in adulthood are offered to adolescents. Laparoscopic gastric banding leads to significant weight loss in childhood and adolescence. A meta-analysis by Paulus et al. (2015) showed a BMI reduction of 11.6 kg/m^2 on average in the first year. Afterwards, no further weight reduction occurred. According to the above meta-analysis, the intraoperative complication rate is very low (bleeding) at 0.8%. Later gastric band-specific complications such as slippage, malfunction and port revisions occurred in this meta-analysis in over 11%, gastrointestinal side effects such

as nausea, vomiting, reflux and diarrhoea in 10%. Vitamin deficiency occurred only in exceptional cases. Regular substitution seems to be not necessary in adolescents. With regard to comorbidities, remission of arterial hypertension, sleep apnea and type 2 diabetes mellitus usually occurs. Quality of life is significantly improved by increased physical activity, improved integration and increased self-confidence. A further advantage of the gastric band is usually the potential reversibility, which should be taken into account especially during childhood and adolescence. Studies on long-term outcome of body weight are not available yet.

There is an increasing shift in bariatric surgery from gastric banding to gastric bypass and sleeve gastrectomy, even in children and adolescents.

Weight loss is most pronounced in gastric bypass surgery, as shown by the meta-analysis of Paulus et al. (2015). After 10 years there is an "excess body weight loss" of 78% according to a retrospective study by Nijhawan et al. (2012). Perioperative complications occur in 5%. These include anastomotic leak and bleeding. Late complications are described in 20% of cases. These are mainly obstructions, internal hernias and ulcers. Gastrointestinal side effects include nausea, vomiting and—particularly worth mentioning—the so-called dumping syndrome. Sometimes in-patient stays are necessary due to dehydration and nutrient deficiencies. The decisive factor is that, in contrast to gastric banding, vitamin and trace element deficiencies occur more frequently, so that regular supplementation is necessary. Comorbidities are significantly reduced after a gastric bypass surgery. The quality of life of young people also improved.

There are only a few studies available on the use of a sleeve gastrectomy especially in children and adolescents. The weight loss due to this surgical procedure is comparable to that of gastric bypass surgery. The intraoperative complication rate is very low and is reported in the meta-analysis as less than 1%.

In the study by Alqahtani et al. (2012), over 90% of patients experienced remission or improvement of comorbidities within 2 years after sleeve gastrectomy. Vitamin and trace element deficiencies rarely occurred. The quality of life also improved significantly.

All three surgical procedures lead to significant weight loss in morbidly obese adolescents.

Due to the scarce data, further studies are needed to assess the long-term consequences with regard to physical and mental development in childhood and adolescence. In 2015, seven active studies were registered in ▶ ClinicalTrials.gov, which investigate the effect of bariatric surgery in adolescents. In a prospective study by Inge et al. (2016), in which 242 adolescents underwent bariatric surgery, a significant weight loss as well as a reduction of comorbidities was shown over a period of 3 years. However, vitamin and trace element substitution were necessary occasionally; in particular iron deficiency and vitamin B_{12} deficiency occurred.

> **Practical Tip**
>
> Until further long-term results are available, bariatric surgery in childhood and adolescence is reserved for individual cases only, despite good results.

16.3 High Risk Patients

A precise definition of high-risk patients does not exist. Ultimately, weight in itself is a risk factor and, in the very high range with BMI > 60 kg/m^2, can lead to the patient becoming a high-risk patient simply because of this. Obesity-related comorbidities, above all pronounced obstructive sleep apnea or other cardiopulmonary concomitant diseases, can quickly lead to the patient becoming a high-risk patient.

There are no study-based recommendations regarding bariatric surgery in this patient group. Bariatric surgery should not be ruled out prematurely in a high-risk patient. Patients with concomitant cardiopulmonary diseases, transplanted patients, but also patients with chronic diseases may be eligible for bariatric surgery. Bariatric surgery often leads to a significant improvement in the health status of these patients due to weight loss. In liver and kidney transplant patients, there is an improvement in organ function, pulmonary hypertension or hypertensive heart disease improves, and sometimes the use of home oxygen is no longer necessary. Bariatric surgery is often the only alternative for these patients, as conservative therapy programs cannot achieve the desired success due to immobility.

Preoperatively, an optimisation of the therapy of the underlying diseases, sometimes also on an inpatient basis, should be aimed at. The operation should be carried out in specialised centres that have the necessary infrastructure with regard to the underlying and concomitant diseases. Malabsorptive procedures are contraindicated in immunocompromised patients or in patients who are permanently taking NSAIDs, in these cases gastric banding or sleeve gastrectomy is preferred.

For high-risk patients, the use of a stepwise approach should be considered. This includes an in-patient caloric restriction, then the subsequent placement of a gastric balloon for further preoperative weight reduction. Due to technical limitations, a restrictive procedure in the form of a sleeve gastrectomy usually takes place as a first operation and, after further weight reduction, the malabsorptive procedure is performed as the second operation if this is still necessary.

> **Practical Tip**
>
> It should be noted that bariatric surgery can be performed on high-risk patients, especially if the associated weight reduction can improve the underlying disease.

References

Alqahtani AR, Antonisamy B, Alamri H et al (2012) Laparoscopic sleeve gastrectomy in 108 obese children and adolescents aged 5–21 years. Ann Surg 256:266–273

Huang CK, Garg A (2015) Bariatric Surgery in old age: a comparative study of laparoscopic Roux-en-Y gastric bypass and sleeve gastrectomy in an Asia centre of excellence. J Biomed Res 29:118–124

Inge TH, Courcoulas AP, Jenkins TM et al (2016) Weight loss and health status 3 years after bariatric surgery in adolescents. N Engl J Med 374:113–123

Kromeyer-Hauschild WM, Kunze D et al (2001) Perzentile für den Body Mass Index für das Kindes- und Jugendalter unter Heranziehung verschiedener deutscher Stichproben. Monatsschr Kinderheilk 8:807–818

Musella M, Milone M, Maietta P et al (2014) Bariatric surgery in elderly patients. A comparison between gastric banding and sleeve gastrectomy with five years of follow up. Int J Surg 12(Suppl. 2): S69–S72

Nijhawan S, Martinez T, Wittgrove AC (2012) Laparoscopic gastric bypass for the adolescent patient: long-term results. Obes Surg 22:1445–1449

Paulus GF et al (2015) Bariatric surgery in morbidly obese adolescents: a systematic review and metaanalysis. Obes Surg 25:860–878

Qin C, Luo B (2014) Advanced age as an independent predictor of perioperative risk after laparoscopic sleeve gastrectomy. Obes Surg 25:406–412

Sugerman HJ, DeMaria EJ, Kellum JM, et al (2004) Effects of bariatric surgery in older patients. Ann Surg. 240:243–247

Treadwell JR, Sun F, Schoelles K (2008) Systematic review and metaanalysis of bariatric surgery for pediatric obesity. Ann Surg 248:763–776

Wabitsch M (2014) Adipositas. In: Hoffmann GF, Lentze MJ, Spranger J (Hrsg) Pädiatrie. Springer, Heidelberg

Further Readings

Abdullah A, Wolfe R, Stoelwinder JU et al (2011) The number of years lived with obesity and the risk of all-cause and cause-specific mortality. Int J Epidemiol 40:985–996

Al Mohaidly M, Suliman A, Malawi H (2013) Laparoscopic sleeve gastrectomy for a two- and half year old morbidly obese child. Int J Surg Case Rep 4: 1057–1060

Al-Qahtani AR (2007) Laparoscopic adjustable gastric banding in adolescent: safety and efficacy. J Pediatr Surg 42:894–897

Angrisani L, Favretti F, Furbetta F et al (2005) Obese teenagers treated by Lap-Band System: the Italian experience. Surgery 138:877–881

Deutsche Gesellschaft für Allgemein- und Viszeralchirurgie, Chirurgische Arbeitsgemeinschaft für Adipositastherapie (CAADIP), Deutsche Adipositas-Gesellschaft (DAAG), Deutsche Gesellschaft für Psychosomatische Medizin und Psychotherapie, Deutsche Gesellschaft für Ernährungsmedizin (2010) S3-Leitlinie: Chirurgie der Adipositas. http://www.adipositas-gesellschaft.de/fileadmin/PDF/Leitlinien/ADIP-6-2010.pdf. (25. April 2016)

Dietz WH, Robinson TN (1998) Use of the body-mass-index (BMI) as a measure of overweight in children and adolescents. J Pediatr 132:191–193

Fatima J, Houghton SG (2006) Bariatric surgery at the extremes of age. J Gastrointest Surg 10:1392–1396

Fried M, Yumuk V, Oppert J-M et al (2013) Interdisciplinary European guidelines on metabolic and bariatric surgery. Obes Facts 6:449–468

Gesundheitsberichterstattung des Bundes 05.02.2015. www.gbe-bund.de (19.07.2016)

Himes JH, Dietz WH (1994) Guidelines for overweight in adolescent preventive services: recommendations from an expert committee. Am J Clin Nutr 59: 839–846

International Pediatric Endosurgery G (2009) IPEG guidelines for surgical treatment of extremely obese adolescents. J Laparoendosc Adv Surg Tech A 19(Suppl. 1):xiv–xvi

Micozzi MS, Albanes D, Jones DY, Chumlea WC (1986) Correlations of body-mass-index with weight, stature, and body composition in men and women in NHANES I and II. Am J Clin Nutr 44:725–731

Nadler EP, Youn HA, Ren CJ et al (2008) An update on 73 US obese pediatric patients treated with laparoscopic adjustable gastric banding: comorbidity resolution and compliance data. J Pediatr Surg 43:141–146

Nadler EP, Barefoot LC, Qureshi FG (2012) Early results after laparoscopic sleeve gastrectomy in adolescents with morbid obesity. Surgery 152:212–217

Oude Luttikhuis H, Baur L, Jansen H et al (2009) Interventions for treating obesity in children. Cochrane Database Syst Rev (1):CD001872

Peraglie C (2015) Laparsocopic mini-gastric bypass in patients age 60 and older. Surg Endosc 30:38–43

Pietrobelli A, Faith MS, Allison DB, Gallagher D, Chiumello G, Heymsfeld SB (1998) Body-mass-index as a measure of adiposity among children and adolescents: a validation study. J Pediatr 132:204–210

Silberhumer GR, Miller K, Pump A et al (2011) Long-term results after laparoscopic adjustable gastric banding in adolescent patients: follow-up of the Austrian experience. Surg Endosc 25:2993–2999

Thereaux J, Poitou C (2014) Midterm outcomes of gastric bypass for elderly (aged ≥ 60 yr) patients: a comparative study. Surg Obes Relat Dis 11:836–841

Yitzhak A, Mizrahi S, Avinoach E (2006) Laparoscopic gastric banding in adolescents. Obes Surg 16: 1318–1322

Obesity Centre

R. Weise

Contents

© Springer-Verlag GmbH Germany, part of Springer Nature 2022
J. Ordemann, U. Elbelt (eds.), *Obesity and Metabolic Surgery*,
https://doi.org/10.1007/978-3-662-63227-7_17

Adiposity centres at large municipal hospitals or university clinics usually have all the necessary disciplines under one roof. In contrast, obesity centres in smaller, partly rural hospitals often have to rely on external cooperation partners. In these centres with a large catchment area, aftercare can also be organised close to home at external locations. Both concepts are possible and can show comparably good long-term results

17.1 Establishment and Certification of an Obesity Centre

The establishment of an obesity centre must be very well prepared. It has been proved to be a good idea to present and discuss the topic of adiposity, metabolic disorders and treatment methods in detail at the so-called round table. Employees from as many hospital departments as possible should participate (▶ Overview: "Recommended Employees and Departments"). This is the only way to reduce frequent prejudices against the future patients. In addition, such a round table is best suited for brainstorming, listing equipment deficiencies and constructional deficits and later eliminating those.

Recommended Employees and Departments for an Internal Round Table
- Surgery with the involvement of nursing and operating personnel
- Internal medicine with the involvement of nursing staff
- Psychosomatics with the involvement of nursing staff
- Medical and nursing staff of the intensive care unit
- Nursing service management
- Administration

- Physiotherapy
- Case manager
- Controlling
- Nutrition/kitchen
- Building services

Since in Germany the performance of metabolic interventions is not yet part of the service obligation of the statutory health insurances (Gesetzlichen Krankenversicherungen, GKV), prior information of the most important cost units and the responsible medical service can help to reduce time-consuming inquiries. Of course, the extension of the range of services offered by the clinic should be mentioned and negotiated with the cost bearers as part of budget negotiations.

The German Society for General and Visceral Surgery (Deutsche Gesellschaft für Allgemein- und Viszeralchirurgie, DGAV) has defined the personal requirements for surgeons and the structures in the hospital to obtain certification as a centre for obesity surgery. According to these certification regulations, it is possible to apply for certification as a centre of competence, reference or excellence. The individual certification levels differ to a large extent regarding the numbers of operations and the increasing demand to publish scientific papers.

The currently valid version of the certification regulations can be viewed and downloaded from the DGAV website (▶ www.dgav.de).

17.2 Interdisciplinary Treatment Team: Obesity Board

From the indication to the treatment of late complications after a metabolic intervention, the cooperation of many medical disciplines is necessary. In addition to a close cooperation

17

between surgeons and internists, a close cooperation with specialists in psychosomatics/psychiatry is equally important. For example, there is a strong association between obesity and psychopathic abnormalities (see also ► Sect. 1.6).

Since a large proportion of the patients affected suffer from metabolic disorders, specialists in endocrinology and diabetology are indispensable cooperation partners in the treatment of obesity. From initial contact to long-term aftercare, qualified nutritional advice plays a decisive role.

In addition, other specialist disciplines often have to be consulted in individual cases. In some cases, an individual treatment concept must be agreed with pulmonologists and cardiologists. Furthermore, the sequence of joint-replacing and bariatric interventions must be determined with orthopaedic surgeons.

Practical Tip

It is advisable to set up a meeting of an interdisciplinary obesity board at regular intervals to discuss indications and complications and to establish individual treatment plans. Obesity conferences are a prerequisite for certification of the obesity centre.

A special role is played by family doctor care close to home. A family doctor who does not know or accept the principles of treating obese patients can only treat bariatric patients inadequately. Here, the holding of regular information events can be helpful.

17.3 Necessary Hospital Equipment

The equipment of the clinic must be consistently adapted to the needs of obese patients, starting with the sufficient size of the surgical shirts and ending with the sufficient load-bearing capacity of the sanitary facilities.

◘ Table 17.1 Necessary equipment of an obesity clinic

Scales	Minimum load 300 kg, sufficient number
Seating facilities	Sufficiently wide, possibly without armrests, up to 300 kg loadable chairs and benches in the waiting areas, examination rooms and patient rooms
Patient beds/ examination couches	Sufficient dimensions, heavy-duty gallows, high load capacity, easy to move
Surgical shirts	Oversized surgical shirts may have to be specially made
Duvets	Sufficiently wide and long plumes
Patient toilets	Minimum load 300 kg, this also applies to the mobile commode chairs of the stations
Patient lift	Occasionally a patient lift with sufficient load capacity is necessary
Blood pressure cuffs	Incorrectly dimensioned blood pressure cuffs result in incorrect blood pressure values, therefore oversize must be present
Operating tables	Sufficiently loadable operating tables, which can still be adjusted under load

◘ Table 17.1 lists the most important minimum requirements that should be present in an obesity clinic.

17.4 Multimodal Treatment Processes

The implementation of conservative multimodal treatment procedures should be covered by the obesity centre. The indications and the multimodal therapy itself are described elsewhere (► Sect. 2.6).

In addition to centre-specific treatment programs, supra-regional multimodal treatment concepts are also available (◘ Table 17.2).

◘ **Table 17.2** Examples of multimodal therapy concepts in Germany

Name of the program	Institution responsible	Contact details
Vivantes Vital	Zentrum für Adipositas und Metabolische Chirurgie, Vivantes Klinikum Spandau, Berlin, Germany	► www.adipositaszentrum.berlin
Obesity Balance	Interdisciplinary Obesity Centre—Charité, Berlin	► www.adipositaszentrum-berlin.de
MMK	Multimodal therapy concept—Diakoniekrankenhaus Henriettenstift, Hannover	► www.adipositaschirurgie-hannover.de
Phoenix Program	Adipositas-Zentrum Nord-West—St. Marien-Hospital, Friesoythe	► www.adipositaszentrum-nord-west.de
Adi Posi Fit	Sana Adiposity Centre NRW—Remscheid	► www.sana-adipositas-nrw.de
DOC WEIGHT®	Federal Association of German Nutritional Physicians	► www.bdem.de
M.O.B.I.L.I.S.	M.O.B.I.L.I.S.—Freiburg	► www.mobilis-programm.de
OPTIFAST®	Nestlé HealthCare Nutrition GmbH—Frankfurt/Main	► www.optifasthome.de

17.5 Self-Help Groups and Internet Portals

Self-help groups (SHG) are an ideal bridge between the patients and the specialist institutions of an obesity centre. Here people with the same problems can meet, exchange information and help each other. For these reasons, every obesity centre should endeavour to promote the establishment and maintenance of at least one obesity SHG in its catchment area. However, in any support, care should be taken to ensure that the SHG retains its independence and autonomy toward the obesity centre.

New participants can inform themselves about treatment options and the effects of a bariatric procedure. In this way, they learn beyond the professional consultation what they are getting involved in and what to expect. Many SHGs support their members in applying for reimbursement and certify their participation in the monthly meetings.

The SHGs always provide the obesity centre with the opportunity to inform its patients about innovations and changes. In addition, joint events and lectures by the various disciplines of the obesity clinic strengthen the bond and create trust.

In addition to the self-help groups, the internet presence of the obesity centre is an important source of information. Many patients and relatives of affected persons inform themselves about the disease and treatment options of obesity with the help of the internet and often choose the clinic of their choice based on the internet presence.

In addition, information brochures and events can be published and, if necessary, posted on social networks (Facebook, Twitter, etc.).

General practitioners are also increasingly obtaining information through these media.

17

17.6 Patient Presentations and Information Material

The level of information of patients with obesity is often insufficient at the time of first presentation. Since the treatment of obesity and its accompanying diseases can be very complex on the one hand and on the other hand due to the extreme changes in behaviour and nutrition, detailed information and counselling measures are necessary.

Appropriate brochures can help to convey basic knowledge and clear up misunderstandings. In addition, lectures can interactively impart the essential treatment topics and offer the opportunity to answer and discuss questions. These measures should contain the following information:

- Basic knowledge about the disease obesity and its accompanying diseases,
- Information on operational procedures, including their risks, realistic prognosis and long-term effects,
- Alternative concepts of treatment,
- Behavioural and nutritional concepts after surgical interventions,
- Education about lifelong aftercare, including the need for lifelong substitution of food supplements.

The "b.m.i.-circle" was developed for this purpose under the auspices of the Bundesverband Deutscher Ernährungsmediziner e. V. (Federal Association of German Nutritionists). This bariatric multimodal information program (b.m.i.) consists of 7 modules that cover all important topics concerning bariatric surgery and its long-term effects.

Modules of the "b.m.i.-Circle"

1. Behaviour: Test of courage—self-care
2. Surgery: Under the knife
3. Nutrition: From liquid to solid
4. Nutritional medicine: Where is the journey heading
5. Nutrition/behaviour: Training Camp Eating Behaviour
6. Behaviour/SHG: We are not alone
7. Nutrition: Enjoy for life

The "b.m.i.-circle" provides for a training course prior to the performance of a bariatric intervention, in which the modules are taken at intervals of 1–2 weeks (i.e. a total of 6–12 weeks preparation time before the operation). The program, including the training material, can be viewed and obtained on the internet portal of the German Nutritional Medical Association (▶ www.bdem.de).

In addition to the regular lectures mentioned above, larger annual information events have proven to be a good idea. These "open house days" serve to exchange information and are generally very well received. Patients, relatives, family doctors and specialists can get to know the entire obesity team of a centre. Additional topics can be offered by other disciplines through lectures, presentations and information desks, for example from

- Plastic surgery,
- Physical therapy,
- Obesity SHGs,
- Companies with auxiliary products,
- Pharmacies.

17.7 Treatment and Patient Pathways

Taking into account quality requirements, necessary process optimizations and required transparency, it is possible to map all treatment steps from the initial presentation to follow-up care in treatment paths. The creation of these pathways, in which employees from all responsible departments should be involved, requires considerable time and effort. However, the very creation of these pathways usually leads to process optimization. Checklists, which are placed at suitable process intersections, can fill the treatment pathways with life.

A treatment pathway (patient pathway) should also be created specifically for individual patients, informing them about the timing of their treatment (timeline).

Further Readings

Berg A, König D (2011) Vorteile körperlicher Aktivität bei der Gewichtsreduktion. Adipositas 5:3–9

Cousins JH, Rubovits DS, Dunn JK, Reeves RS, Ramirez AG, Foreyt JP (1992) Family versus individually oriented intervention for weight loss in Mexican American women. Public Health Rep 10:549–555

Deutsche Adipositas-Gesellschaft, Deutsche Diabetes Gesellschaft, Deutsche Gesellschaft für Ernährung, deutsche Gesellschaft für Ernährungsmedizin (2014) Interdisziplinäre Leitlinie der Qualität S3 zur "Prävention und Therapie der Adipositas". AWMF-Register Nr. 050/001. Klasse: S3. Version 2.0. http://www.adipositas-gesellschaft.de/fileadmin/PDF/Leitlinien/S3_Adipositas_Praevention_Therapie_2014.pdf. (25. April 2016)

König D, Berg A (2012) Bewegung als Therapie bei Diabetes mellitus Typ 2. Internist 53:678–687

Paul-Ebhohimhen V, Avenell A (2009) A systematic review of the effectiveness of group versus individual treatments for adult obesity. Obes Facts 2:17–24

17

Alternative Techniques and Methods in Obesity Therapy

C. A. Jacobi

Contents

© Springer-Verlag GmbH Germany, part of Springer Nature 2022
J. Ordemann, U. Elbelt (eds.), *Obesity and Metabolic Surgery*,
https://doi.org/10.1007/978-3-662-63227-7_18

18.1 **Gastric Plication**

The good results after sleeve resection led to the development of another surgical procedure that uses the principle of restriction without resecting a large part of the stomach. This so-called gastric plication is performed laparoscopically, like all bariatric operations.

The stomach is first dissected at the large curvature as in sleeve resection and all vessels up to the left diaphragm are cut through. In contrast to the sleeve, a reverse suture is then applied (◘ Fig. 18.1). Several rows of sutures are necessary to achieve sufficient restriction. As in sleeve gastrectomy, a gastric tube is required to calibrate the lumen. Despite the lack of standardization in the choice of suture material, most authors recommend non-resorbable suture materials of the thickness 2.0–3.0. Both single-button as well as continuous sutures are described.

The main mechanism of action of gastric plication is the achieved restriction. In contrast to sleeve gastrectomy, ghrelin-producing cells are not removed, so ghrelin production is not affected. Furthermore, vagal nerve fibres, which are partially dissected in sleeve gastrectomy or gastric bypass, remain unaffected. Neurohumoral effects as a result of this partial dissection are therefore not achieved by gastric plication.

Various authors describe this operation as being easily performed and, with a low complication rate, as safe and effective. Possible complications are gastric perforations and bleeding. Furthermore, insufficient weight loss has been described.

The indication for surgery corresponds to that of established surgical procedures. Some authors recommend this method on the one hand especially for patients with low morbid obesity, but on the other hand also for patients with very severe obesity. Prospective randomized studies on the long-term effectiveness of gastric plication are still pending. The short-term results published so far show an overall

◘ **Fig. 18.1** Technique of gastric replication by surgery

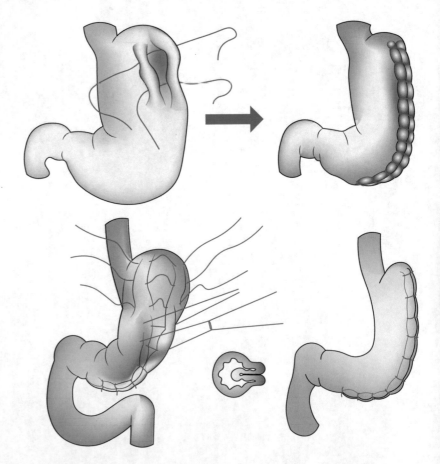

18

significantly lower proportion of patients who achieve an overweight loss comparable to the established procedures. As a possible advantage for the performance of gastric surgery, some authors mention the lower operation costs, since no stapler devices are required. However, the presumed higher rate of revision surgery in cases of insufficient weight loss must be taken into account.

The possible combination with other bariatric surgical procedures has also been described for gastric plication. For example, a gastric band can be implanted proximally to the plication to prevent dilatation of the stomach and to achieve greater effectiveness in terms of weight loss over the long term.

A final assessment of the value of the gastric ligature can therefore not yet be made.

18.2 POSE Procedure

The POSE procedure is a complete endoluminal procedure. The stomach is endoscopically gathered intra-luminally, thus creating a restriction comparable to the gastric plication. For this demanding procedure a specially developed equipment is required. So far, only preliminary clinical results are available for this method. It should be noted that a standardized calibration by means of a gastric tube is not possible.

Possible advantages of the method are the outpatient feasibility of the procedure, the avoidance of skin incisions and the absence of the need for general anaesthesia with intubation. The duration of this procedure in analgo-sedation is comparable to that of established laparoscopic surgical procedures. However, the fact that endoscopic procedures in the stomach and the esophagus have not been established in the therapy of reflux diseases and the results described in the literature are not satisfactory remains to be criticized. The procedure is strongly advertised by the manufacturers of the necessary accessories, but it remains unclear whether the method will establish itself and for which patient groups it will be used. In addition, the costs for the user and the reimbursement by the health insurances have not yet been clarified.

18.3 Endobarrier®

The endoscopic application of the Endobarrier™ uses the principle of eliminating food intake in the duodenum and the first part of the jejunum resulting in missing hormonal changes. The chyme passes an endoluminally placed tube system with its fixation in the area of the pylorus (◻ Fig. 18.2), so that the intestinal mucosa of the duodenum and

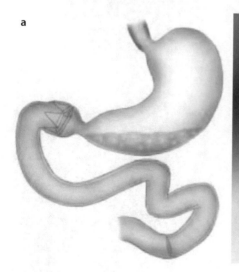 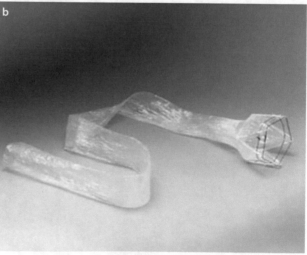

◻ **Fig. 18.2   a, b** Endoscopic gastric bypass (Endobarrier™ with inlay). A plastic tube (inlay, **b**) is anchored postpylorically and thus a functional elimination of the duodenum is achieved. The results obtained so far are promising, the significance in the overall concept is still unclear. (From Wirth and Hauner 2013)

upper jejunum do not come into contact with the food. Preliminary results on the implantation of an Endobarrier™ mainly refer to the technique, complications and short-term results. A weight loss that is reached with the established surgical procedures cannot be achieved by this procedure. However, the effects on glucose regulation in patients with diabetes mellitus type 2 are remarkable. However, a remission without additional drug therapy of diabetes mellitus type 2 remains an exception.

The Endobarrier™ is an alternative for patients who are sceptical about or reject surgery. As with all procedures, an additive multimodal therapy should be applied especially in this procedure. Furthermore, patients must be informed about the necessity of replacement or removal of the system after 12 months at the latest. There is no acceptance of this procedure by the health insurance so far, therefore an individual application has to be made. A recommendation of this system for general use is not given by the European Network for Health Technology in Health Care (EUnetHTA) due to the described complications.

18.4 Gastric Sleeve with Ileum Interposition

Another experimental bariatric surgical procedure, which is mainly used in obese patients with existing diabetes mellitus type 2, is the gastric sleeve formation with postpyloric ileum interposition (◘ Fig. 18.3).

In this endoscopic procedure, a gastric sleeve resection is performed first. Then the post-pyloric cut of the duodenum 2–3 cm behind the pylorus is done with a forklift truck and the stomach is moved to the lower abdomen. After locating the Treitz ligament, the jejunum is marked 50 cm aborally with a suture. This is the intended site of connection of the ileum loop to be interposed. The identification of the terminal ileum and cecum follows. Thirty centimeter in front of the

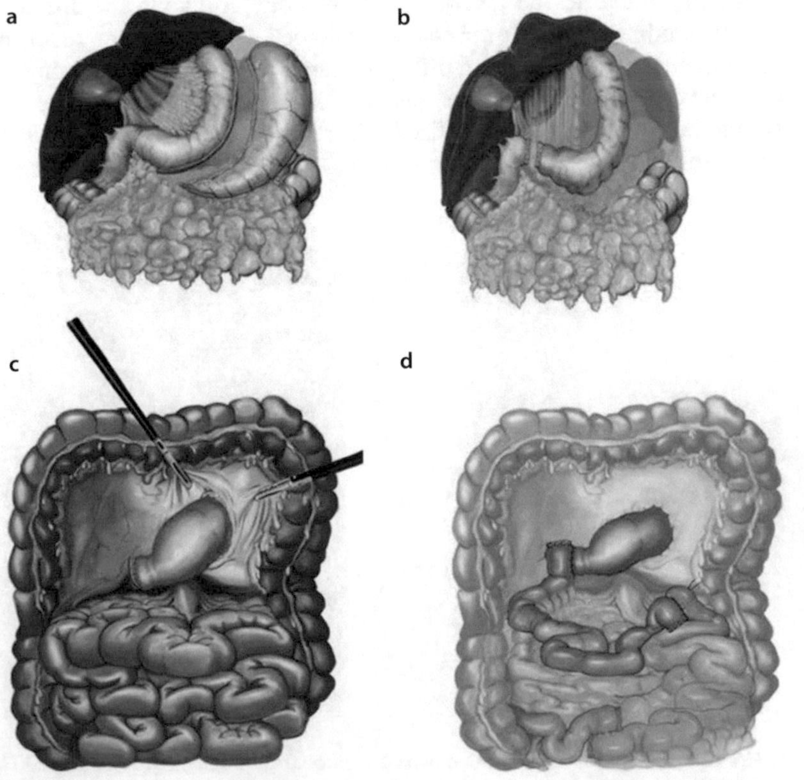

◘ **Fig. 18.3** **a–d** Gastric sleeve formation with postpyloric ileum interposition. (From Celik et al. 2015)

Bauhin's valve a 170 cm long piece of ileum is dissected and relocated to the middle abdomen. Subsequently, anastomosis of the interponate to the jejunum 50 cm behind the Treitz ligament and anastomosis to the duodenum are performed. Additionally, the area of the resected ileum segment is anastomosed. Thus, three anastomoses are necessary, which can be applied either by hand suture or mechanically with a stapler device. The presumed mechanism of this operation consists of a direct influence of gastrointestinal hormones in addition to the restriction through the gastric sleeve. The present studies mainly deal with the perioperative complications and the postoperative short-term results.

One of the largest series was published by Celik's research group (Celik et al. 2015). 360 patients at an average age of 51 years were operated on, in whom the HbA_{1c} was 9.4% on average. The complication rate was high (6.1%), almost 2% of the patients had to undergo emergency revision. The average BMI reduction was 28%. Results on HbA_{1c}-reduction were not reported. Therefore, the significance of this operation cannot yet be conclusively assessed.

18.5 Securing Different Operation Procedures with a Band or a Ring

The use of a ring or band in the proximal portion of a gastric sleeve or on the pouch of a bypass is not new. However, in recent years more and more different products have been introduced to the market, which are increasingly used in the clinic. The so-called Fobi-Ring, the GaBP-Ring™ and the Minimizer™ are available. The principles of these products are based on mechanistic thinking. The additional placement of a ring or band is intended to prevent dilatation of the distal parts of the stomach or intestine (□ Fig. 18.4). The placement of a ring or band can be used for the primary placement of a gastric bypass or a tubular stomach. After bariatric surgery with consecutive dilatation, the ring or band can also be placed during a second operation.

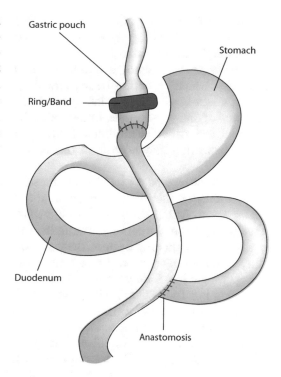

□ **Fig. 18.4** Bypass with ring reinforcement to prevent dilatation

Favourable long-term results are available for the primary application of a band for gastric bypass as well as for sleeve resection. In a study published by Lemmens et al. (2014) with a small number of patients with complete follow-up, the average overweight loss after a banded bypass was 85% after 4 years. Further prospective randomized studies are still needed. The additional costs for the ring systems are not yet covered by health insurance companies.

Additional complications, such as the migration of these systems to the gastric wall, must be considered and communicated to the patient during the explanation.

18.6 Gastric Stimulator

Gastric stimulation as a further experimental procedure has been used for several years in the treatment of obesity. There is no clearly defined indication. With a gastric stimulator (VBloc™, EnteroMedics) approved by the American regulatory authority FDA for the treatment of obesity, patients with a BMI between 35 and 45 kg/m^2 achieved a 24% loss of overweight after 18 months.

The system consists of a pacemaker and electrodes, which can often be implanted on an outpatient basis. By stimulating or blocking fibres of the vagus nerve, hunger and the feeling of satiety can be modified. Restriction or malabsorption play no role in this procedure.

In a review by Cha et al. (2014), the results of 31 studies on this subject are summarised and analysed. Although the authors conclude that electrical stimulation of the stomach can be a successful therapy option, there are no data for such a conclusion. For example, the average weight loss is only small and therefore the indication for patients with a very high BMI is not given. In addition, most follow-up intervals are short and no conclusions can be drawn about the long-term effect. Therefore, the future and more studies on this topic will show if this cost-intensive procedure with a rather low overweight loss can become established.

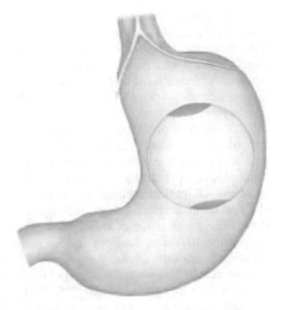

☐ **Fig. 18.5** Gastric balloon. The filling volumes of the mostly water-filled balloons are 400–700 ml. The S3 guideline sees its importance especially for high-risk patients (e.g. BMI > 60 kg/m^2) within the framework of a step-by-step concept. (From Wirth and Hauner 2013)

patients to undergo established bariatric surgical procedures after weight loss.

18.7 Gastric Balloon

Another possible intervention for short-term weight loss before a planned bariatric procedure is the implantation of a gastric balloon. During a gastroscopy, the balloon is inserted in an empty state and then filled with up to 700 ml of fluid (☐ Fig. 18.5). This results in an indirect restriction with an increased feeling of satiation, so that a weight reduction of approximately 20% of the overweight can be achieved. After 6 months at the latest, the stomach balloon must be removed endoscopically. Usually, the patient regains weight rapidly after removal of the gastric balloon, so that the gastric balloon placement as an isolated method does not lead to good long-term results with regard to weight loss. Furthermore, the costs of the implantation are usually not covered by the insurance companies. Within the framework of a step-by-step concept for the treatment of obesity, however, the implantation of a gastric balloon might be useful to enable selected high-risk

18.8 AspireAssist™

Another experimental procedure is the AspireAssist™. This is a type of PEG probe that is inserted into the stomach during gastroscopy and the end of the probe is pulled through the abdominal wall to the outside. The patient then has the opportunity to suck it out or drain it with a hand pump about 20 min after a meal.

This system is indicated for patients with a BMI between 35 and 55 kg/m^2. Possible acute complications correspond to those of PEG-attachment (bleeding, malfunction, perforation, infection, dislocation). Results from clinical studies are rare. In a publication by Sullivan et al. (2013) 11 patients were treated with this system as well as additive nutritional counselling and lifestyle intervention. No complications were documented within 2 years. The reduction of overweight was about 50%. The application of this system remains controversial for a variety of reasons.

18

References

Celik A, Ugale S, Ofluoglu H, et al (2015) Technical feasibility and safety profile of laparoscopic diverted sleeve gastrectomy with ileal transposition (DSIT). Obes Surg. 25: 1184–90

Cha R, Marescaux J, Diana M (2014) Updates on gastric electrical stimulation to treat obesity: systematic review and future perspectives. World J Gastrointest Endosc 6:419–431

Lemmens L, Karcz WK, Bukhari W, Fink J, Kuesters S (2014) Banded gastric bypass—four years follow up in a prospective multicenter analysis. www.biomedcentral.com/1471-2482/14/88

Sullivan S, Stein R, Jonnalagadda S, Mullady D, Edmundowicz S (2013) Aspiration therapy leads to weight loss in obese subjects: a pilot study. Gastroenterology 145:1245–1252

Wirth A, Hauner H (eds) (2013) Adipositas. Springer, Berlin, Heidelberg

Further Readings

Broderick RC, Fuchs HF, Harnsberger CR, Sandler BJ, Jacobsen GR (2014) Comparison of bariatric restrictive operations: laparoscopic sleeve gastrectomy and laparoscopic gastric greater curvature plication. Surg Technol Int 25:82–89

Colquitt JL, Pickett K, Loveman E, Frampton GK (2014) Surgery for weight loss in adults. Cochrane Database Syst Rev 8:CD003641

Daigle CR, Corcelles R, Schauer PR (2015) Primary silicone-banded laparoscopic sleeve gastrectomy: a pilot study. J Laparoendosc Adv Surg Tech A 25:94–97

Fobi MA, Lee H, Felahy B, Che-Senge K, Fields CB, Sanguinette MC (2005) Fifty consecutive patients with the GaBP ring system used in the banded gastric bypass operation for obesity with follow up of at least 1 year. Surg Obes Relat Dis 1:569–572

Iannelli A, Amato D, Addeo P et al (2008) Laparoscopic conversion of vertical banded gastroplasty (Mason MacLean) into Roux-en-Y gastric bypass. Obes Surg 18:43–46

Lee WJ, Lee KT, Ser KH, Chen JC, Tsou JJ, Lee YC (2015) Laparoscopic adjustable gastric banding (LAGB) with gastric plication: short-term results and comparison with LAGB alone and sleeve gastrectomy. Surg Obes Relat Dis 11:125–130

Lewis MC, Phillips ML, Slavotinek JP, Kow L, Thompson CH, Toouli J (2006) Change in liver size and fat content after treatment with Optifast very low calorie diet. Obes Surg 16:697–701

Nausheen S, Shah IH, Pezeshki A, Sigalet DL, Chelikani PK (2013) Effects of sleeve gastrectomy and ileal transposition, alone and in combination, on food intake, body weight, gut hormones, and glucose metabolism in rats. Am J Physiol Endocrinol Metab 305:507–518

Talebpour A, Heidari R, Zeinoddini A, Talebpour M (2015) Predictors of weight loss after laparoscopic gastric plication: a prospective study. J Laparoendosc Adv Surg Tech A 25:177–181. https://doi.org/10.1089/lap.2014.0193

Tessa V, Givan F, Mathus-Vliegen E, Veldhuyzen E, Conchillo J, Bouvy N, Fockens P (2015) Endoscopic gastric volume reduction with a novel articulating plication device is safe and effective in the treatment of obesity. Gastrointest Endosc 81:312–320

Zechmeister-Koss I, Huić M, Fischer S, European Network for Health Technology Assessment (EUnetHTA) (2014) The duodenal-jejunal bypass liner for the treatment of type 2 diabetes mellitus and/or obesity: a systematic review. Obes Surg 24:310–323

Supplementary Information

Index

Printed in the United States
by Baker & Taylor Publisher Services